THE IMPROVED IBS DIET AND GUIDE FOR BEGINNERS

A COMPREHENSIVE ELIMINATION DIET PLAN FOR FAST RELIEF FROM IRRITABLE BOWEL SYMPTOMS

Copyright © 2024 Aashvi Dhingra

All rights reserved.

THE IMPROVED IBS DIET AND GUIDE FOR BEGINNERS 1
INTRODUCTION: WHAT IS IBS ALL ABOUT? 2
    Type of IBS: Constipation-Predominant, Diarrhea-Predominant, Mixed 2
    Signs and Symptoms of IBS 5
    Causes and Risk Factors 6
    Differentiating IBS from Other Digestive Disorders 8
    Medications for Symptom Relief: Antispasmodics, Antidiarrheals, Laxatives 9
Getting Started with the IBS Elimination Diet 11
    Historical Context and Evolution of Elimination Diets in IBS Management 11
    How Does an Elimination Diet Work? 12
    Comparisons with Other Dietary Approaches 14
    Different Approaches to Elimination Diets 17
    Sequential Elimination vs. Simultaneous Elimination 18
4 WEEKS ELIMINATION PROTOCOL 18
30 DAYS ELIMINATION DIET MEAL PLAN 21
Chapter 1: Vegan and Vegetarian Recipes for IBS 24
    Quinoa Salad and Tahini Dressing 25
    Lentil Soup and Spinach 27
    Chickpea and Vegetable Curry 29
    Tofu Stir-Fry and Tamari Sauce 31
    Black Bean Tacos with Corn Tortillas 33
    Rice Noodle and Soy Sauce 35

Hummus and Veggie Wrap 37
Stuffed Bell Peppers and Corn 39
Vegan Chili with Kidney Beans 41
Falafel Bowl and Mediterranean Salad 43
Caprese Salad with Tomato 45
Vegetable Frittata with Spinach 47
Grilled Portobello Mushroom Burger 49
Eggplant Parmesan and Vegan Cheese 51
Spinach and Ricotta Stuffed Pasta Shells 53
Vegetable Pad Thai with Tofu 55
Vegetarian Sushi Rolls and Carrot 58
Roasted Vegetable Pizza and Red Onion 60
Veggie Wrap with Goat Cheese 62
Quinoa Stuffed Acorn Squash 64

GLUTEN-FREE AND DAIRY-FREE OPTIONS 66
Grilled Salmon with Steamed Vegetables 67
Quinoa Salad with Roasted Vegetables 69
Chicken, Vegetable Stir-Fry and Brown Rice 71
Baked Chicken Breast and Sautéed Spinach 73
Shrimp and Avocado Salad 75
Turkey Meatballs with Spaghetti Squash 77
Lentil Soup with Carrots and Kale 79
Grilled Steak with Roasted Brussels Sprouts 81
Chickpea and Basmati Rice 83
Vegetable Stir-Fry with Broccoli 86
Gluten-Free Pasta with Tomato Basil Sauce 88
Turkey and Vegetable Chili 90
Baked Cod and Quinoa Pilaf 92
Eggplant and Zucchini Lasagna 95
Spinach with Gluten-Free Toast 97
Tofu and Vegetable Pad Thai 99
Vegan Buddha Bowl and Tahini Sauce 101

    Roasted Vegetable Salad and Balsamic Glaze 103
    Turkey and Gluten-Free Tortilla 105
    Quinoa Stuffed Bell Peppers and Salsa 107
Poultry, Meat and Potatoes 109
    Grilled Chicken and Roasted Potatoes 110
    Turkey Chili and Crushed Tomatoes 112
    Baked Turkey Meatballs and Spaghetti Squash 114
    Lemon Herb Roasted Chicken Thighs 116
    Chicken, Stir-Fry and Brown Rice 118
    Turkey and Vegetable Soup 120
    Grilled Turkey Burger 122
    Chicken Caesar Salad and Dairy-Free Dressing 124
    Turkey and Avocado Wrap 126
    Turkey and Vegetable Kabobs 128
    Grilled Steak and Mashed Sweet Potatoes 130
    Beef with Broccoli 132
    Beef and Bean Chili 134
    Lamb Kebabs and Quinoa Tabbouleh 136
    Beef and Mushroom Stroganoff 139
    Beef and Cabbage Soup 141
    Pork Tenderloin with Roasted Root Vegetables 143
    Meatloaf and Steamed Green Beans 145
    Beef and Basmati Rice 147
    Pork Stir-Fry with Bell Peppers 149
    Baked Potato and Steamed Broccoli 151
    Mashed Potatoes 153
    Roasted Potato Wedges and Herbs 155
    Potato Salad with Dijon Mustard Dressing 157
    Sweet Potato Hash with and Spinach 159
    Potato and Leek Soup 161
    Scalloped Potatoes and Yeast 163

    Hasselback Potatoes with Rosemary 165
    Potato Pancakes 167
    Potato and Vegetable Frittata 169

IBS friendly Breakfast and Brunch Recipes 171
    Scrambled eggs with spinach 172
    Grilled chicken salad and olive oil vinaigrette 174
    Night Prepared Oats 176
    Turkey and avocado lettuce wraps 178
    Smoothie and protein powder 180
    Quinoa salad with chickpeas 181
    Greek yogurt parfait with berries 183
    Turkey and vegetable soup 185
    Omelet with mushrooms 187
    Quinoa and black bean salad 189
    Smoothie bowl and pumpkin seeds 191
    Chicken with tamari sauce 192
    Chia seed pudding with berries 194
    Lentil and vegetable soup 196

IBS friendly Dinner Options 198
    Baked salmon and quinoa 199
    Stir-fried tofu and brown rice 201
    Grilled shrimp skewers and marinara sauce 203
    Baked chicken breast and mashed sweet potatoes 205
    Grilled steak with roasted asparagus 207
    Baked cod and wild rice 209
    Turkey meatballs and marinara sauce 211

IBS Friendly Desserts and Sweet Treats 213
    IBS Fruit Salad 214
    Dark Chocolate 216
    Banana Nice Cream 218
    Oatmeal Cookies 220
    Coconut Yogurt Parfait 222

  Rice Pudding..228
  Peanut Butter Energy Balls 230
  Baked Apples..232
  Almond Flour Blueberry Muffins.....................................234
References..236
Appendices..242
  Food Lists: High FODMAP Foods, Low FODMAP Foods..242
    Low FODMAP Pantry Staples: 246
SYMPTOMS TRACKING JOURNAL..248
REINTRODUCTION SYMPTOMS ASSESSMENT 256
Conversion Charts 264
RECIPE INDEX..265

INTRODUCTION: WHAT IS IBS ALL ABOUT?

Irritable Bowel Syndrome (IBS) is a common gastrointestinal disorder characterized by a cluster of symptoms affecting the digestive system. It is a chronic condition that affects the lifestyle of those suffering from it. IBS is considered a functional gastrointestinal disorder, meaning it affects how the digestive system works without causing any visible damage or abnormalities. Functional GI disorders, now termed disorders of gut-brain interactions by doctors, involve issues with the coordination between your brain and your gut. These issues can result in increased gut sensitivity and alterations in bowel muscle contractions. Heightened gut sensitivity can lead to increased abdominal pain and bloating, while changes in bowel muscle contractions can cause diarrhea, constipation, or both.

Type of IBS: Constipation-Predominant, Diarrhea-Predominant, Mixed

Irritable Bowel Syndrome (IBS) is a heterogeneous condition, meaning it can manifest in various ways with different predominant symptoms. The major known types are the constipation-predominant IBS/IBS-C, diarrhea-predominant IBS/IBS-D, and mixed IBS/IBS-M. Understanding the differences between these subtypes is crucial for accurate diagnosis and effective management.

Constipation-Predominant IBS (IBS-C):

Individuals with IBS-C primarily experience symptoms related to constipation. This includes infrequent bowel movements, difficulty passing stools, and a feeling of incomplete evacuation. If you have the IBS-C; on days when you have at least one abnormal bowel movement, more than a quarter of your stools are hard or lumpy and less than a quarter of your stools are loose or watery. The underlying mechanisms contributing to constipation in IBS-C may involve abnormalities in gastrointestinal motility, decreased colonic transit time, and altered sensation in the gut. Management strategies for IBS-C often focus on increasing fiber intake, hydration, regular exercise, and the use of laxatives or stool softeners to promote bowel regularity and alleviate symptoms.

Diarrhea-Predominant IBS (IBS-D):

IBS-D is characterized by frequent episodes of diarrhea, loose or watery stools, urgency to have a bowel movement, and an increased frequency of bowel movements. If you are diagnosed with IBS-D; on days when you have at least one abnormal bowel movement, more than a quarter of your stools are loose or watery and less than a quarter of your stools are hard or lumpy. Possible underlying mechanisms contributing to diarrhea in IBS-D include abnormal gut motility, increased intestinal permeability, and alterations in the gut microbiota. Management of IBS-D often involves dietary modifications, such as avoiding trigger foods and incorporating low-FODMAP diet, as well as medications such as antidiarrheals, antispasmodics, and gut-targeted medications like rifaximin.

Mixed IBS (IBS-M):

Mixed IBS is characterized by the presence of both constipation and diarrhea symptoms, often alternating between the two. Individuals with IBS-M may experience periods of constipation followed by episodes of diarrhea or vice versa. When you've the IBS-M type; on days when you have at least one abnormal bowel movement, more than a quarter of your stools are hard or lumpy and more than a quarter of your stools are loose or watery. The alternating nature of symptoms in IBS-M can significantly impact an individual's quality of life and may require a tailored approach to management. Treatment strategies for IBS-M may involve a combination of interventions targeting both constipation and diarrhea symptoms, such as dietary modifications, fiber supplementation, and medications to regulate bowel function.

And lastly, recent interactions with several people who noticed symptoms related to IBS but yet struggle with healing or getting relief have revealed some possible cause; and if you are experiencing such, this is what you can do going forward:

The cause of your problems may be full or partial bowel dysmotility; this is particularly true if you do not respond to dietary changes (high fiber) or medication (especially prescriptions). The first step in treating your problems is to have colonic inertia tested; other tests that are recommended are those that check for small bowel dysmotility, pelvic floor problems, rectal problems, and slow emptying of the stomach (gastroparesis). All of these tests should be part of a routine work-up. If your GI doesn't do it, you should look for a neurogastroenterologist and visit a motility clinic, which are few but do exist. You can find one online and at most teaching hospitals.

Signs and Symptoms of IBS

Irritable Bowel Syndrome (IBS) is characterized by a range of signs and symptoms that can vary widely among individuals. While the presentation of IBS can differ from person to person, there are several common symptoms associated with the condition.

Abdominal Pain: One of the hallmark symptoms of IBS is abdominal pain or discomfort. This pain is often described as cramping, sharp, or dull and may occur anywhere in the abdomen. The intensity and frequency of abdominal pain can vary, ranging from mild and intermittent to severe and persistent.

Bloating: Many individuals with IBS experience bloating, which is a feeling of fullness or swelling in the abdomen. Bloating can be accompanied by visible distension of the abdomen and may worsen throughout the day, particularly after eating certain foods or meals.

Gas: Increased gas production is another common symptom of IBS. This may manifest as excessive belching or flatulence (passing gas). Gas-related symptoms can contribute to abdominal discomfort and bloating in individuals with IBS.

Diarrhea: Diarrhea is a prevalent symptom in some individuals with IBS, particularly those with diarrhea-predominant IBS (IBS-D). It is characterized by loose or watery stools, increased frequency of bowel movements, and urgency to defecate. Diarrhea episodes may be triggered by certain foods, stress, or other factors.

Constipation: Conversely, constipation is a common symptom in others, especially those with constipation-predominant IBS (IBS-C). Constipation is characterized by infrequent bowel movements, difficulty passing stools, and a feeling of incomplete evacuation. Individuals with IBS-C may also experience straining during bowel movements.

The variability and severity of symptoms in IBS can fluctuate over time, with periods of remission where symptoms are minimal or absent, followed by flare-ups where symptoms worsen. Factors such as stress, diet, hormonal changes, and underlying gastrointestinal abnormalities can influence the frequency and intensity of symptoms. The symptoms tracker on page 246 will help you keep a tab on food triggers.

Causes and Risk Factors

The development of Irritable Bowel Syndrome (IBS) is believed to be influenced by a combination of factors, including various potential contributors and triggers. Understanding these causes and risk factors is crucial for managing the condition effectively.

Women are up to two times more likely than men to develop IBS. People younger than age 50 are more likely to develop IBS than people older than age 50.

Factors that can increase your chance of having IBS include:

Diet: Dietary factors play a significant role in IBS, with certain foods and beverages known to trigger or exacerbate symptoms in susceptible individuals. Common dietary triggers include high-fat foods, spicy foods, dairy products, caffeine, alcohol, and foods high in fermentable carbohydrates known as FODMAPs. These foods can contribute to the different symptoms experienced by IBS patients.

Stress: Psychological stress is closely linked to the onset and exacerbation of IBS symptoms. Stressful life events, anxiety, and depression can significantly impact gut function and increase susceptibility to gastrointestinal symptoms. The gut-brain axis, a bidirectional communication system between the gut and the brain, plays a key role in this relationship, with stressors affecting gut motility, sensitivity, and immune function.

Gut Microbiota: The gut microbiota, comprising trillions of microorganisms residing in the gastrointestinal tract, plays a critical role in gut health and function. Imbalances or alterations in the composition and diversity of gut bacteria, known as dysbiosis, have been implicated in the development of IBS. Dysbiosis may contribute to inflammation, altered gut motility, and visceral hypersensitivity, leading to the onset or exacerbation of IBS symptoms.

Genetics: Genetic factors are thought to contribute to the susceptibility to IBS, although the precise genetic mechanisms remain unclear. Family and twin studies have provided evidence of a genetic component in IBS, suggesting that certain genetic variations may increase the risk of developing the condition. However, IBS is considered a multifactorial disorder, with genetic predisposition interacting with environmental and lifestyle factors in its pathogenesis.

Read more on the science behind the causes and risk factors of IBS from research papers listed in the reference section.

Triggers and aggravating factors can exacerbate IBS symptoms and precipitate flare-ups in susceptible individuals. Common triggers include:

Dietary Triggers: Consumption of trigger foods such as those high in FODMAPs, spicy foods, or fatty foods can provoke gastrointestinal symptoms in individuals with IBS.

Stress and Anxiety: Emotional stress, anxiety, and other psychological factors can trigger or worsen IBS symptoms by disrupting gut-brain communication and exacerbating gut motility and sensitivity.

Changes in Routine: Disruptions to routine, such as travel, changes in sleep patterns, or alterations in daily activities, can trigger IBS symptoms in some individuals.

Hormonal Changes: Fluctuations in hormone levels, particularly in women during menstruation, pregnancy, or menopause, can influence gut function and exacerbate IBS symptoms.

Medications: Certain medications, such as antibiotics, nonsteroidal anti-inflammatory drugs (NSAIDs), and some antidepressants, may worsen gastrointestinal symptoms in individuals with IBS.

Differentiating IBS from Other Digestive Disorders

Differentiating Irritable Bowel Syndrome (IBS) from other digestive disorders is essential for accurate diagnosis and appropriate management. While IBS shares some similarities with other conditions, there are key differences that help distinguish it from inflammatory bowel disease (IBD), celiac disease, food intolerances, and functional dyspepsia.

Comparison with Inflammatory Bowel Disease (IBD)

IBS and IBD are both chronic gastrointestinal conditions, but they have distinct characteristics and underlying mechanisms. IBD, which includes Crohn's disease and ulcerative colitis, is characterized by chronic inflammation and damage to the digestive tract. Unlike IBS, which is considered a functional disorder with no visible signs of damage, IBD involves identifiable structural abnormalities and inflammatory changes in the gastrointestinal tract, as seen on imaging studies and biopsies. Symptoms of IBD may include abdominal pain, diarrhea (often bloody), weight loss, fatigue, and fever, which can be more severe and persistent than those of IBS. Diagnosis of IBD typically involves endoscopic procedures, imaging studies, and laboratory tests to assess inflammation markers and confirm the presence of structural abnormalities.

Celiac Disease

Celiac disease is an autoimmune disorder triggered by gluten ingestion in genetically susceptible individuals. Like IBS, celiac disease can cause gastrointestinal symptoms such as abdominal pain, bloating, gas, diarrhea, and constipation. However, celiac disease is characterized by an immune-mediated reaction to gluten, leading to damage to the small intestine's lining and malabsorption of nutrients. Diagnosis of celiac disease involves blood tests to detect specific antibodies and confirmation with a small intestine biopsy showing characteristic changes.

Food Intolerances

Food intolerances, such as lactose intolerance or fructose malabsorption, can cause symptoms similar to those of IBS, including bloating, gas, diarrhea, and abdominal pain. Unlike IBS, which is a functional disorder, food intolerances result from the body's inability to digest certain foods due to enzyme deficiencies or other metabolic abnormalities. Diagnosis of food intolerances may involve dietary elimination trials, breath tests, and other diagnostic tests to identify specific food triggers.

Functional Dyspepsia

Functional dyspepsia is another functional gastrointestinal disorder characterized by chronic or recurrent upper abdominal pain or discomfort, often accompanied by early satiety, bloating, nausea, or belching. While some symptoms overlap with IBS, functional dyspepsia primarily affects the upper gastrointestinal tract, whereas IBS predominantly affects the lower gastrointestinal tract. Diagnosis of functional dyspepsia is based on symptom assessment and exclusion of other gastrointestinal conditions through clinical evaluation and diagnostic tests.

Medications for Symptom Relief: Antispasmodics, Antidiarrheals, Laxatives

Medications play a crucial role in managing the symptoms of Irritable Bowel Syndrome (IBS) by targeting specific symptoms such as abdominal pain, diarrhea, and constipation. Several classes of medications are commonly used to provide relief from IBS symptoms, including antispasmodics, antidiarrheals, and laxatives.

Antispasmodics: Antispasmodic medications help alleviate abdominal pain and cramping associated with IBS by relaxing smooth muscle in the gastrointestinal tract.

Commonly prescribed antispasmodics include:

- Hyoscyamine (Levsin)

- Dicyclomine (Bentyl)

- Mebeverine (Colofac)

These medications work by blocking the action of acetylcholine, a neurotransmitter that stimulates smooth muscle contraction in the gut. Antispasmodics are particularly beneficial for individuals with IBS who experience frequent or severe abdominal pain or cramping.

Antidiarrheals: Antidiarrheal medications are used to reduce the frequency and urgency of bowel movements in individuals with diarrhea-predominant IBS (IBS-D).

The most commonly used antidiarrheals for IBS include:

- Loperamide (Imodium)

- Diphenoxylate/atropine (Lomotil)

These medications work by slowing down intestinal motility and increasing the absorption of water and electrolytes in the colon, resulting in firmer stools and decreased diarrhea. Antidiarrheals can provide effective short-term relief from diarrhea symptoms in IBS but should be used cautiously and under medical supervision to avoid potential complications such as constipation or bowel obstruction.

Laxatives: Laxatives are medications used to relieve constipation by promoting bowel movements and softening stools.

In individuals with constipation-predominant IBS (IBS-C), laxatives can help alleviate symptoms such as infrequent bowel movements and difficulty passing stools.

Types of laxatives commonly used for IBS include:

- Bulk-forming laxatives (e.g., psyllium, methylcellulose)

- Osmotic laxatives (e.g., polyethylene glycol, lactulose)

- Stimulant laxatives (e.g., senna, bisacodyl)

These medications work by increasing stool bulk, drawing water into the colon, or stimulating intestinal contractions to facilitate bowel movements. Laxatives should be used judiciously and in accordance with healthcare provider recommendations to prevent dependence and minimize potential side effects such as electrolyte imbalances or dehydration.

Getting Started with the IBS Elimination Diet

The IBS elimination diet is a dietary approach aimed at identifying and eliminating specific foods that may trigger or exacerbate symptoms in individuals with Irritable Bowel Syndrome (IBS). The primary purpose of the elimination diet is to help pinpoint potential dietary triggers and alleviate gastrointestinal symptoms. The elimination diet involves temporarily removing certain foods or food groups from the diet and then gradually reintroducing them one at a time while monitoring for symptom recurrence. By systematically eliminating and reintroducing foods, individuals can identify which foods trigger their symptoms and make informed dietary choices to manage their IBS more effectively.

Historical Context and Evolution of Elimination Diets in IBS Management

Elimination diets have long been used as a therapeutic approach for managing gastrointestinal disorders, including IBS. The concept of dietary modification to alleviate gastrointestinal symptoms dates back centuries, with historical records documenting the use of specific diets to treat digestive ailments.

In the context of IBS management, the concept of elimination diets has evolved over time with advances in scientific research and our understanding of the relationship between diet and gastrointestinal health. Early elimination diets for IBS often involved restricting common trigger foods such as dairy, gluten, and high-fat or spicy foods based on anecdotal evidence and clinical experience.

However, the development of the low-FODMAP diet represents a significant milestone in the evolution of elimination diets for IBS management.

The low-FODMAP diet, initially pioneered by researchers at Monash University in Australia, involves eliminating high-FODMAP foods from the diet for a period of time and then systematically reintroducing them while monitoring symptoms. This evidence-based approach has been shown to be effective in reducing symptoms in a significant proportion in individuals with IBS, particularly those with symptoms related to bloating, gas, and diarrhea.

In recent years, the popularity of the low-FODMAP diet has grown, and it has become widely recognized as a first-line dietary intervention for IBS management. However, it's important to note that the elimination diet approach is not a one-size-fits-all solution, and individual responses to specific foods can vary.

How Does an Elimination Diet Work?

The elimination process involves several key principles aimed at identifying and eliminating foods that may be contributing to gastrointestinal symptoms in individuals with conditions such as Irritable Bowel Syndrome (IBS).

The Principle of Identifying and Eliminating Trigger Foods are;

Elimination Phase: During the elimination phase, certain foods or food groups known to commonly trigger symptoms are removed from the diet for a specified period of time. Common trigger foods for IBS include high-FODMAP foods (e.g., certain fruits, vegetables, legumes, dairy products), gluten-containing grains, spicy foods, caffeine, and alcohol. The duration of the elimination phase may vary but typically ranges from 2 to 6 weeks.

Symptom Monitoring: Throughout the elimination phase, individuals carefully monitor their symptoms and keep track of any changes or improvements in gastrointestinal symptoms such as abdominal pain, bloating, gas, diarrhea, or constipation. Keeping a food and symptom diary can help identify patterns and correlations between specific foods and symptom occurrence.

Reintroduction Phase: After the elimination phase, individual foods or food groups are systematically reintroduced into the diet, one at a time, in small quantities. The reintroduction phase allows individuals to assess their tolerance to specific foods and identify which ones trigger symptoms. Foods are reintroduced gradually, with a waiting period of 2 to 3 days between each new food to allow for symptom assessment.

Symptom Assessment: During the reintroduction phase, individuals closely monitor their symptoms following the reintroduction of each food. If symptoms recur or worsen after reintroducing a particular food, it is considered a potential trigger, and further testing may be warranted to confirm its role in symptom development.

Personalized Approach: The elimination diet is highly individualized, and the specific foods eliminated and reintroduced may vary based on an individual's symptoms, dietary preferences, and suspected trigger foods. Healthcare providers or dietitians may provide guidance and support throughout the process to ensure safe and effective implementation of the elimination diet.

Potential Mechanisms of Symptom Relief

The elimination diet may provide symptom relief in individuals with IBS through several potential mechanisms:

Reduced Gut Irritants: By eliminating trigger foods that may irritate the gastrointestinal tract or contribute to inflammation, the elimination diet helps reduce the overall burden on the digestive system, leading to fewer symptoms.

Balanced Gut Microbiota: Certain foods eliminated during the elimination phase, such as high-FODMAP foods, may feed pathogenic bacteria in the gut and disrupt the balance of the gut microbiota. By removing these foods temporarily, the elimination diet may promote a healthier balance of gut bacteria, which can improve gut health and reduce symptoms.

Improved Gut Barrier Function: Some foods eliminated during the elimination phase, such as gluten or certain additives, may contribute to increased intestinal permeability (leaky gut) in susceptible individuals. Removing these potential triggers may help restore gut barrier function and reduce the passage of harmful substances into the bloodstream, leading to symptom relief.

Identification of Individual Triggers: The reintroduction phase of the elimination diet allows individuals to identify specific foods that trigger their symptoms, enabling them to make informed dietary choices and avoid future symptom flare-ups. This personalized approach to dietary management can lead to long-term symptom relief and improved quality of life for individuals with IBS.

Comparisons with Other Dietary Approaches

While elimination diets, particularly the low-FODMAP diet, have shown efficacy in managing IBS symptoms, they are not the only dietary approach available. Other dietary strategies for managing IBS include:

High-Fiber Diet

First off, there are two kinds of fiber;

- Insoluble fiber - this kind of fiber speeds up your digestive track and adds more liquid to the equation - this is bad for anyone suffering from ibs or other stomach issues.

- Soluble fiber - this fiber slows down your digestive tract giving it more time to properly digest and absorb nutrients. This is good. It absorbs excess water while at the same time providing a solid gel like substance which helps cause "normality" in your bowels. This is good whether your problem is that you go too much or not enough. A high-fiber diet, particularly soluble fiber, may benefit individuals with IBS by promoting regular bowel movements and improving stool consistency.

The problem here is that food in general does not contain very much soluble fiber. Things like berries, whole grains, vegetables, other fruits and other high fiber foods contain large quantities of the bad insoluble and low quantities of the good soluble essentially offsetting each other.

So, you've got to supplement soluble fiber.

Trust me, go to the store and buy a plain unflavored no sugar or anything added container of fiber. There should only be one ingredient: soluble fiber. Any artificial sweeteners and chemicals will just upset your gut further and the plain flavor tastes fine in water. Also, the store brand is fine there is no need to pay double or more for brand name supplements. Don't listen to the instructions on the label.

For severe cases take two full tablespoons with a full glass of water each. One tablespoon in the morning and one at night. For mild cases just take one tablespoon at night. The morning dose may cause more gas throughout the day which you don't want if you don't have to.

Make sure to increase your water consumption accordingly, not doing this will cause problems. Read up on how much you should be drinking for your size.
This does not work instantly, you will notice a small difference within the first week and huge improvements after a month or less.

Probiotics

Probiotics are beneficial bacteria that may help restore gut microbiota balance and alleviate symptoms in individuals with IBS. While the evidence for probiotics in IBS management is mixed, some individuals may experience symptom improvement with specific strains of probiotics.

Gluten-Free Diet

Some individuals with IBS may benefit from a gluten-free diet, particularly those with non-celiac gluten sensitivity. Eliminating gluten-containing grains such as wheat, barley, and rye may reduce symptoms in susceptible individuals.

Mindful Eating

Mindful eating practices, such as paying attention to hunger and fullness cues, chewing food thoroughly, and eating in a relaxed environment, may help individuals with IBS better manage their symptoms by promoting optimal digestion and reducing stress-related symptoms.

Furthermore, there are tons of diets and suggestions out there. But that's because IBS isn't a disease; it's a syndrome. That basically means that it's a group of similar symptoms exhibited by people where the root cause and treatment are not entirely known. Some people get diarrhea, others get constipated. What works for me, probably won't work for you. You need to work with your doctor and experiment on your own to find the best overall diet and treatment that's right for you.

Therefore we cannot have a one size fits all approach to manage or cure this as it has to be very individualistic , this is why most allopathic doctors will simply put you on antibiotics or proton pump inhibitors that will be helpful in the short term but there will be a relapse once you stop taking them. And every time there is a relapse it gets worse because you're wiping off the healthy bacteria in your gut microbiome and also developing antibiotic resistance to an extent.

IBS can be managed and healed. Several people have experienced permanent relief by following what I'm about to share with you, but the treatment needs to be individualistic or it causes more damage than good.

However I will share some proven information that will be helpful for anyone suffering from IBS as per documented testimonies:

Long term IBS is directly associated with nutrient depletion and your body's ability to manufacture and process nutrients. Therefore it is important to supplement with Vitamin B Complex (make sure it has B1,B3 ,B5,B6,B12 in bioavailable forms)

Vitamin D3 is extremely important for various metabolic functions regulating circadian rhythms and assisting your immune response. It's important to supplement with at least 5000 iu daily for 30–60 days to get to optimum levels.

IBS and damaged gut lining are inter related which means, 99% of IBS patients have a leaky gut. Supplement with 5 grams of L-Glutamine twice a day to start healing your gut lining.

Different Approaches to Elimination Diets

Different approaches to elimination diets include specific elimination protocols targeting common trigger foods and customized dietary modifications tailored to individual symptoms and preferences.
Specific Elimination Diets:

Low FODMAP Diet

The low FODMAP diet focuses on reducing intake of fermentable carbohydrates known as FODMAPs. High-FODMAP foods can exacerbate symptoms in individuals with IBS by increasing fermentation and gas production in the gut. The low FODMAP diet involves eliminating high-FODMAP foods during the elimination phase and gradually reintroducing them to identify trigger foods.

Gluten-Free Diet

A gluten-free diet eliminates foods containing gluten, a protein found in wheat, barley, rye, and their derivatives. For individuals with gluten sensitivity or celiac disease, consuming gluten-containing foods can trigger gastrointestinal symptoms and damage the intestinal lining. Eliminating gluten-containing grains and products can alleviate symptoms and promote gut healing in susceptible individuals.

Dairy-Free Diet

A dairy-free diet excludes dairy products such as milk, cheese, yogurt, and butter. Some individuals may be lactose intolerant, unable to digest lactose, the sugar found in dairy products, leading to symptoms such as abdominal pain, bloating, and diarrhea. Removing dairy from the diet can provide relief from gastrointestinal symptoms in lactose-intolerant individuals.

Sequential Elimination vs. Simultaneous Elimination

Elimination diets can be implemented using either sequential elimination or simultaneous elimination approaches:

Sequential Elimination: In sequential elimination, individual foods or food groups are eliminated one at a time, and symptoms are monitored before moving on to the next elimination phase. This approach allows for systematic identification of trigger foods and simplifies the reintroduction process.

Simultaneous Elimination: Simultaneous elimination involves removing multiple potential trigger foods or food groups from the diet at once. While this approach may expedite the identification of trigger foods, it can be more challenging to pinpoint specific triggers and may increase the risk of nutritional deficiencies if not carefully planned.

4 WEEKS ELIMINATION PROTOCOL

A 4-week elimination protocol is a structured dietary approach designed to identify and eliminate potential trigger foods that may exacerbate gastrointestinal symptoms. This protocol involves eliminating specific foods or food groups from the diet for a designated period, followed by a systematic reintroduction phase to identify trigger foods and customize a long-term dietary plan. Here's how a typical 4-week elimination protocol may be structured:

Week 1: Preparation and Elimination

- Preparation: The process kicks off when you start by familiarizing yourself with the elimination protocol guidelines and identify foods or food groups to be eliminated based on your symptoms, dietary history, and potential trigger foods. Make use of the meal plans and recipes in this cookbook during the elimination phase. Take inventory of your current food supplies and identify any high-risk foods or ingredients that need to be eliminated from your diet during the elimination phase. Remove these foods from your pantry, refrigerator, and kitchen to avoid accidental consumption. Learn how to read food labels to identify potential sources of trigger ingredients in packaged foods. Look for hidden sources of gluten, lactose, and other problematic ingredients that may be present in processed or packaged foods.

- Elimination: Start the elimination phase by removing identified trigger foods from your diet completely. Common trigger foods may include gluten-containing grains, dairy products, high-FODMAP foods, caffeine, alcohol, spicy foods, and processed or high-fat foods. Focus on consuming whole, minimally processed foods that are allowed on the elimination protocol, such as lean proteins, fruits, vegetables, gluten-free grains, and dairy-free alternatives.

Weeks 2-3: Maintenance and Symptom Tracking

- Consistency: Maintain the elimination diet rigorously throughout weeks 2 and 3 to ensure accurate assessment of symptom changes and identify potential trigger foods. Avoid consuming any foods or ingredients that are not allowed on the elimination protocol, and be mindful of cross-contamination and hidden sources of trigger ingredients in packaged or processed foods.

- Symptom Tracking: Keep a detailed food and symptom diary to track your dietary intake and any changes in gastrointestinal symptoms. Record the foods you eat, portion sizes, preparation methods, and any symptoms experienced, including their severity and duration. Regularly assess your symptoms and look for patterns or correlations between specific foods or meals and symptom occurrence.

Week 4: Reintroduction and Evaluation

- Reintroduction: The reintroduction phase starts with the systematic reintroduction of eliminated foods or food groups, one at a time, while monitoring for symptom recurrence. Start with small portions of the reintroduced food and gradually increase the serving size over several days while you observe any changes in symptoms. Reintroduce foods that are most likely to be tolerated first, such as those with lower likelihood of triggering symptoms.

- Symptom Evaluation: Monitor your symptoms closely after reintroducing each food, paying attention to any changes or exacerbation of symptoms. Keep track of the specific food reintroduced, portion size, and any symptoms experienced. Allow a few days between reintroductions to ensure accurate assessment of symptom response.

- Customization: Customize your long-term dietary plan based on the identified trigger foods, your individual tolerance, and nutritional needs.

- Monitoring and Adjustment: Regularly monitor your symptoms and dietary intake to ensure ongoing symptom management and make adjustments to your dietary plan as needed. Be open to revisiting the elimination protocol periodically to reassess your tolerance to trigger foods and make further modifications if necessary.

30 DAYS ELIMINATION DIET MEAL PLAN

WEEK 1	BREAKFAST	LUNCH	DINNER
DAY 1	Scrambled eggs with spinach	Grilled chicken salad and olive oil vinaigrette	Baked salmon and quinoa
DAY 2	Overnight oats	Turkey and avocado lettuce wraps	Stir-fried tofu and brown rice
DAY 3	Smoothie and protein powder	Quinoa salad with chickpeas	Grilled shrimp skewers and marinara sauce
DAY 4	Greek yogurt parfait with berries	Turkey and vegetable soup	Baked chicken breast and mashed sweet potatoes
DAY 5	Omelet with mushrooms	Quinoa and black bean salad	Grilled steak with roasted asparagus
DAY 6	Smoothie bowl and pumpkin seeds	Chicken and tamari sauce	Baked cod and wild rice
DAY 7	Chia seed pudding with	Lentil and vegetable soup	Turkey meatballs and

	berries		marinara sauce

Week 2: Repeat meals from Week 1, or try new recipes with similar ingredients.

Week 3 and 4: Keep eating a variety of meals that concentrate on healthy foods and steer clear of ingredients that trigger your food intolerance, just as in Weeks 1 and 2. To spice up your dishes, try using various herbs, spices, and cooking techniques.

MAIN TOPIC: MEAL IDEAS AND IBS FRIENDLY RECIPES

Chapter 1: Vegan and Vegetarian Recipes for IBS

(Choose Low FODMAP Ingredients when necessary; The list in Appendices will guide you).

Quinoa Salad and Tahini Dressing

Serving	Kcal	Carbs	Proteins	Fats	Fiber
4	250	30g	8g	12g	5g

Prep Time: 15 minutes
Cooking Time: 15 minutes
Total Time: 30 minutes

Ingredients

- 1 cup quinoa, rinsed
- 2 cups water or vegetable broth
- 1 cup mixed vegetables diced
- 1/4 cup fresh parsley, chopped
- 1/4 cup fresh mint leaves, chopped

Lemon-Tahini Dressing

- 1/4 cup tahini
- 2 tablespoons lemon juice
- 1 clove garlic, minced
- Salt, pepper, water

Step By Step Preparations

Commence by bringing a medium pot of water or vegetable broth to a boil. Once boiling, add the quinoa, then reduce the heat to low, cover, and allow it to simmer for 15 minutes, or until the quinoa is fully cooked. Remove from heat and let it cool slightly.

Transfer the cooked quinoa to a large mixing bowl along with the mixed veggies, mint, and parsley.

In a separate small bowl, combine the tahini, lemon juice, water, minced garlic, salt, and pepper, whisking until a smooth and creamy consistency is achieved.

Drizzle the lemon-tahini dressing over the quinoa and vegetable mixture. Gently toss everything together until evenly coated. Taste and adjust the seasoning.

This salad goes well with grilled chicken or fish as an addition or as a light meal or supper. For those suffering from IBS, quinoa is an excellent option since it is gluten-free, high-protein, and high-fiber whole grain.

Lentil Soup and Spinach

Serving	Kcal	Carbs	Proteins	Fats	Fiber
4	250	35g	12g	7g	12g

Prep Time: 15 minutes
Cooking Time: 30 minutes
Total Time: 45 minutes

Ingredients

- 1 cup dry green or brown lentils, rinsed and drained
- 4 cups vegetable broth
- 2 carrots, diced
- 2 stalks celery, diced
- 1 cup spinach, chopped
- 2 tablespoons olive oil
- 1 teaspoon ground cumin
- 1 teaspoon ground coriander
- 1/2 teaspoon ground turmeric
- Salt, pepper, fresh lemon wedges

Step by Step Preparations

Heat the olive oil in a big pot over medium heat. Add in and cook the chopped celery and carrots for about five minutes, or until they start to soften. Right after that, add the rinsed lentils to the pot and mix in the vegetable broth, salt, pepper, ground cumin, ground coriander, and powdered turmeric. Once the soup reaches a boiling point, lower the heat to a simmer, cover, and let the soup cook for 20 to 25 minutes, or until the lentils are soft. After the lentils are cooked, add the chopped spinach to the pot and stir until it wilts, which should take about two to three minutes. Taste the soup and add more salt and pepper if you want. Serve hot, with the option to garnish it with fresh lemon wedges to squeeze over it before eating.

You can have this soup as a filling meal by itself, or you can pair it with a side salad or a slice of bread suitable for a low FODMAP diet.

Chickpea and Vegetable Curry

Serving	Kcal	Carbs	Proteins	Fats	Fiber
4	350	30g	9g	22g	8g

Prep Time: 15 minutes
Cooking Time: 25 minutes
Total Time: 40 minutes

Ingredients

- 1 can (15 oz) chickpeas, drained and rinsed
- 1 can (14 oz) coconut milk
- 2 cups bell peppers, zucchini, and green beans, diced
- 1 onion, finely chopped
- 2 cloves garlic, minced
- 1 tablespoon ginger, minced
- 2 tablespoons curry powder
- 1 teaspoon ground cumin
- 1 teaspoon ground coriander
- 1/2 teaspoon turmeric powder
- 1 tablespoon olive oil
- Salt, pepper, fresh cilantro
- Cooked rice or quinoa

Step by Step Preparations

In a large pan or pot, warm the olive oil over medium heat. After adding the chopped onion, sauté it for three to four minutes, or until it becomes transparent. Add the ginger and garlic, minced, and simmer for a further one to two minutes, or until aromatic. Add the turmeric powder, ground coriander, ground cumin, and curry powder and stir. Cook, stirring regularly until the spices are roasted and aromatic. Add the mixed vegetables to the skillet and cook for about 5 minutes, until slightly softened. Then, pour in the coconut milk and stir to combine while you let the mixture simmer. Next, add the chickpeas and stir well to coat them with the coconut milk and spices. Now, let the curry simmer for a further 10 to 15 minutes. Lastly, Season with salt and pepper to taste.

To lessen the symptoms of IBS, choose low-FODMAP veggies like bell peppers, zucchini, and green beans. This curry can be eaten on its own as a light meal or combined with quinoa or rice for a heartier meal.

Tofu Stir-Fry and Tamari Sauce

Serving	Kcal	Carbs	Proteins	Fats	Fiber
4	250	15g	15g	15g	5g

Prep Time: 15 minutes
Cooking Time: 15 minutes
Total Time: 30 minutes

Ingredients

- 1 block (14 oz) firm tofu, pressed and cubed
- 2 bell peppers, sliced
- 2 cups broccoli florets
- 2 tablespoons tamari sauce
- 2 tablespoons sesame oil
- 2 cloves garlic, minced
- 1 tablespoon ginger, minced
- 2 green onions, sliced
- Cooked rice or quinoa

Step by Step Preparations

Tofu should first be wrapped in paper towels and pressed with a heavy object to squeeze out any extra moisture. After 15 minutes, cut the tofu into cubes.

On medium-high heat, warm a big pan or wok with 1 tablespoon of sesame oil. Toss in the cubes of tofu and cook, turning once in a while, for about 5 to 7 minutes, or until they are crispy and golden brown. Put the tofu aside for a second after taking it out of the pan.

Put the last tablespoon of sesame oil into the same pan. Toss in the minced ginger and garlic and sauté for a minute or two, or until they release their aromatic scent.

Then, toss in the broccoli florets and sliced bell peppers to the pan. To make the veggies tender-crisp, stir-fry them for around seven to ten minutes.

Add the cooked tofu and veggies back to the pan. Coat the tofu and veggies evenly with the tamari sauce by pouring it over them and swirling well.

After another two or three minutes of cooking, the flavors will have had time to combine. Once done, remove the pan from heat and garnish the dish with chopped green onions. Serve the delicious stir-fry hot over cooked rice or quinoa

---

You can add your favorite vegetables or protein sources to this adaptable stir-fry. Choose gluten-free soy sauce.

Black Bean Tacos with Corn Tortillas

Serving	Kcal	Carbs	Proteins	Fats	Fiber
4	300	40g	10g	12g	12g

Prep Time: 15 minutes
Cooking Time: 15 minutes
Total Time: 30 minutes

Ingredients

- 1 can (15 oz) black beans, drained and rinsed
- 8 small corn tortillas
- 1 cup salsa
- 1 ripe avocado, sliced
- 1/2 cup shredded lettuce or cabbage
- 1/4 cup chopped fresh cilantro
- Lime wedges

For the Taco Seasoning:

- 1 teaspoon ground cumin
- 1 teaspoon smoked paprika
- 1/2 teaspoon chili powder
- 1/2 teaspoon garlic powder
- 1/4 teaspoon ground coriander
- Salt and pepper

Step by Step Preparations

In a small bowl, combine all the taco seasoning ingredients: ground cumin, smoked paprika, chili powder, garlic powder, ground coriander, salt, and pepper.

On medium heat, warm a non-stick skillet. Add the drained and rinsed black beans to the skillet, along with the taco seasoning. Cook for 5-7 minutes, stirring occasionally, until the beans are thoroughly heated and coated with the seasoning.

While the beans cook, follow package instructions to warm the corn tortillas. To assemble the tacos, place a spoonful of the seasoned black beans onto each warm corn tortilla.

Top the beans with salsa, sliced avocado, shredded lettuce or cabbage, and chopped cilantro. Serve with lime wedges on the side for squeezing over the tacos.

You can personalize these tacos by adding extra toppings like sliced jalapenos, diced tomatoes, or lactose-free yogurt or low-FODMAP sour cream.

Rice Noodle and Soy Sauce

Serving	Kcal	Carbs	Proteins	Fats	Fiber
4	350	45g	15g	12g	5g

Prep Time: 20 minutes
Cooking Time: 15 minutes
Total Time: 35 minutes

Ingredients

- 8 oz rice noodles
- 1 block (14 oz) firm tofu, pressed and cubed
- 2 heads baby bok choy, chopped
- 3 cloves garlic, minced
- 1 tablespoon fresh ginger, minced
- 2 tablespoons low-sodium soy sauce
- 1 tablespoon rice vinegar
- 1 tablespoon sesame oil
- 1 tablespoon olive oil
- Salt, pepper, sesame seeds
- Sliced green onions

Step by Step Preparations

Start by cooking the rice noodles according to the directions on the box. Once they're done, drain them and keep them away for later use.

In a large sized pan or wok, preheat the olive oil over medium-high heat. Proceed to add the cubed tofu, frying until each side acquires a lovely golden brown tone, often about 5-7 minutes. Once done, take the tofu from the pan and put it aside.

In the same pan, add the minced garlic and ginger, allowing them to simmer for 1-2 minutes until their smell fills the air.

Next, add the chopped bok choy to the pan, cooking for 3-4 minutes while turning often, until it wilts down. Reintroduce the cooked tofu to the skillet, with the bok choy. Add the cooked rice noodles, soy sauce, rice vinegar, and sesame oil to the mix. Combine everything well until all ingredients are properly combined and cooked through.

Adjust the seasoning with salt and pepper. Serve the delectable meal hot, garnishing it with sesame seeds and chopped green onion

For those with IBS who are sensitive to gluten or high-FODMAP foods, rice noodles are a low-FODMAP substitute for wheat-based noodles.

Hummus and Veggie Wrap

Serving	Kcal	Carbs	Proteins	Fats	Fiber
2	250	35g	8g	9g	7g

Prep Time: 10 minutes
Cooking Time: 0 min
Total Time: 10 minutes

Ingredients

- 2 large whole wheat or gluten-free tortillas
- 1/2 cup hummus
- 1 small cucumber, thinly sliced
- 1 medium tomato, thinly sliced
- 1 cup lettuce leaves
- Salt and pepper

Step by Step Preparations

Start by placing the tortillas flat on a clean surface. Evenly distribute 1/4 cup of hummus over each tortilla, careful to leave a little border around the borders.

Arrange cucumber slices, tomato slices, and lettuce leaves on top of the hummus, distributing them equally between the two tortillas. Season with salt and pepper.

Fold the bottom edge of each tortilla up over the contents, then fold in the sides, and roll firmly to make a wrap. For ease, split each wrap in half diagonally, and serve immediately.

You can alter this wrap by adding extras like sliced olives, bell peppers, or shredded carrots. Choose romaine or butter lettuce

Stuffed Bell Peppers and Corn

Serving	Kcal	Carbs	Proteins	Fats	Fiber
4	250	45g	10g	3g	10g

Prep Time: 20 minutes
Cooking Time: 35 minutes
Total Time: 55 minutes

Ingredients

- 4 large bell peppers, any color
- 1 cup cooked quinoa
- 1 can (15 oz) black beans, drained and rinsed
- 1 cup corn kernels, fresh, canned, or frozen
- 1/2 cup diced tomatoes, fresh or canned
- 1/2 cup diced red onion
- 2 cloves garlic, minced
- 1 teaspoon ground cumin
- 1/2 teaspoon smoked paprika
- Salt and pepper
- 1/2 cup shredded cheese
- Fresh cilantro

Step by Step Preparations

Start by preheating the oven to 375°F (190°C) and greasing a baking dish big enough to fit the bell peppers in an upright position.

Prepare the bell peppers by cutting off their tops and removing the seeds and membranes. Place them vertically in the oiled baking dish.

In a big mixing bowl, add the cooked quinoa, black beans, corn, diced tomatoes, diced red onion, minced garlic, ground cumin, smoked paprika, salt, and pepper. Thoroughly mix until all ingredients are thoroughly blended.

Spoon the quinoa and black bean mixture liberally into each bell pepper until they are packed to the capacity and slightly overflowing. Gently push down to pack the filler. For extra taste, sprinkle cheese over the top of each filled bell pepper.

Cover the baking dish with foil and bake in the preheated oven for 25 minutes. Then, remove the cover and continue baking for an additional 10 minutes, or until the bell peppers are soft and the mixture is cooked through.

Once done, take the filled bell peppers out of the oven and allow them to cool for a few minutes before serving. garnish with fresh cilantro before serving it boiling hot.

For a dairy-free option, feel free to omit the cheese and add additional veggies or herbs.

Vegan Chili with Kidney Beans

Serving	Kcal	Carbs	Proteins	Fats	Fiber
4	200	30g	8g	6g	10g

Prep Time: 15 minutes
Cooking Time: 30 minutes
Total Time: 45 minutes

Ingredients

- 1 can (15 oz) kidney beans, drained and rinsed
- 1 can (14 oz) crushed tomatoes
- 1 onion, diced
- 2 bell peppers, diced
- 2 cloves garlic, minced
- 1 tablespoon olive oil
- 1 tablespoon chili powder
- 1 teaspoon ground cumin
- 1/2 teaspoon paprika
- Salt, pepper, fresh cilantro
- Sliced green onions
- Dairy-free yogurt or avocado slices

Step by Step Preparations

In a large sized saucepan or Dutch oven, warm up the olive oil over medium heat. Toss in the diced onion and sauté until it softens, 3-4 minutes.

Introduce the minced garlic to the saucepan, simmering for a further 1-2 minutes until it emits its aromatic scent. Incorporate the chopped bell peppers into the saucepan, simmering for around 5 minutes until they begin to soften.

Sprinkle in the chili powder, ground cumin, paprika, salt, and pepper, ensuring the veggies are well covered with the spices as you stir.

Add the crushed tomatoes and kidney beans to the saucepan, stirring well to mix all the ingredients. Allow the chili to achieve a soft simmer, then decrease the heat to low. Cover the saucepan and let the chili simmer for approximately 20-25 minutes, stirring regularly, until the flavors merge together and the chili thickens to your taste.

Taste the chili and adjust the seasoning if required, adding more salt and pepper if preferred. Serve the chili hot, garnishing with fresh cilantro, chopped green onions, dairy-free yogurt, or avocado slices.

Serve it as a stand-alone dish, or as a full meal with a side salad or a slice of low-FODMAP bread

Falafel Bowl and Mediterranean Salad

Serving	Kcal	Carbs	Proteins	Fats	Fiber
4	400	50g	14g	17g	10g

Prep Time: 20 minutes
Cooking Time: 20 minutes
Total Time: 40 minutes

Ingredients

- 1 cup dry quinoa, rinsed
- 2 cups water
- 1 can (15 oz) chickpeas, drained and rinsed
- 2 cloves garlic, minced
- 1/4 cup fresh parsley, chopped
- 1 teaspoon ground cumin
- 1 teaspoon ground coriander
- 1/2 teaspoon ground paprika
- Salt, pepper
- 2 tablespoons olive oil
- Mixed greens or lettuce
- 1 cucumber, diced
- 1 tomato, diced
- 1/4 red onion, thinly sliced
- 1/4 cup Kalamata olives, pitted and halved
- 1/4 cup hummus
- Lemon wedges

Step by Step Preparations

In a medium saucepan, start by mixing the washed quinoa and water. Bring the mixture to a boil, then decrease the heat to simmer, covering it for approximately 15-20 minutes until the quinoa is thoroughly cooked and the water is absorbed. Once done, remove the pot from the heat and fluff the quinoa with a fork.

While the quinoa cooks, make the falafel mixture. In a food processor, mix together the chickpeas, minced garlic, chopped parsley, ground cumin, ground coriander, ground paprika, salt, and pepper until thoroughly blended, but still somewhat chunky.

In a large pan over medium heat, heat 1 tablespoon of olive oil. Form the falafel mixture into small patties or balls and fry them in the pan for 3-4 minutes on each side until they attain a golden brown, crispy finish. Repeat this procedure with the remaining falafel mixture, adding extra olive oil to the pan as required.

As the falafel cooks, create the Mediterranean salad. In a large bowl, mix together the mixed greens or lettuce, diced cucumber, diced tomato, thinly sliced red onion, and halved Kalamata olives until thoroughly incorporated.

To make the falafel bowls, divide the cooked quinoa equally among four bowls. Top each dish with falafel patties, Mediterranean salad, and a liberal dollop of hummus. For additional flavor, serve the falafel bowls with lemon wedges on the side for squeezing over the top.

For those who are lactose intolerant or sensitive to dairy, hummus gives the falafel bowl a creamy texture and an extra protein boost without using dairy products.

Caprese Salad with Tomato

Serving	Kcal	Carbs	Proteins	Fats	Fiber
4	250	5g	15g	20g	1g

Prep Time: 10 minutes
Cooking Time: 0 min.
Total Time: 10 minutes

Ingredients

2 large tomatoes, sliced

8 oz fresh mozzarella cheese, sliced

1/4 cup fresh basil leaves

2 tablespoons extra virgin olive oil

1 tablespoon balsamic vinegar

Salt, pepper

Step by Step Preparations

Begin by arranging the tomato slices and fresh mozzarella slices on a serving platter, alternating between them for a visually appealing presentation.

Tuck fresh basil leaves between the tomato and mozzarella slices to add flavor and color. Drizzle extra virgin olive oil and balsamic vinegar over the salad, and season with salt and pepper to taste.

This salad pairs well with grilled chicken or fish for a full meal, but it's best enjoyed in the summer when tomatoes and basil are in season for their freshest flavor

Vegetable Frittata with Spinach

Serving	Kcal	Carbs	Proteins	Fats	Fiber
4	180	6g	12g	12g	2g

Ingredients

- 6 large eggs
- 1/4 cup lactose-free milk or unsweetened almond milk
- 1 cup fresh spinach, chopped
- 1 cup mushrooms, sliced
- 1/2 cup bell peppers, diced
- 1/2 cup cherry tomatoes, halved
- 1/4 cup green onions, chopped
- 1 tablespoon olive oil
- Salt, pepper, fresh herbs

Step by Step Preparations

Begin by preheating the oven to 350°F (175°C). In a large mixing basin, whisk together the eggs and lactose-free milk until well combined. Season with salt and pepper to taste.

In a large oven-safe skillet, heat the olive oil over medium heat. Cook the mushrooms and bell peppers for 3-4 minutes, until they soften.
Add the chopped spinach to the pan and simmer for an additional 1-2 minutes, or until wilted.

Evenly distribute the egg mixture among the veggies in the skillet. Sprinkle the cherry tomatoes and green onions over top. Cook a frittata on the stove top for 3-4 minutes, or until the edges start to firm.

Place the pan in the preheated oven and bake for 15-20 minutes, or until the frittata has set in the middle with a faint golden tint on top. Once completely cooked, remove the pan from the oven and let the frittata cool for a few minutes before slicing. Before slicing and serving, top the frittata with fresh herbs.

For those who are lactose intolerant, a creamy frittata can be achieved by using unsweetened almond milk or lactose-free milk.

Grilled Portobello Mushroom Burger

Serving	Kcal	Carbs	Proteins	Fats	Fiber
2	150	10g	3g	12g	5g

Prep Time: 10 minutes
Cooking Time: 10 minutes
Total Time: 20 minutes

Ingredients

- 2 large portobello mushrooms, stems removed
- 1 tablespoon olive oil
- 1 tablespoon balsamic vinegar
- Salt, pepper
- 1 avocado, sliced
- 1 tomato, sliced
- 2 lettuce leaves
- 2 gluten-free hamburger buns or lettuce wraps

Step by Step Preparations

First, preheat the grill to a medium-high temperature. Mix the olive oil and balsamic vinegar in a small bowl using a whisk. After applying this mixture to the portobello mushrooms' two sides, season them with salt and pepper.

Place the mushrooms on the grill, gill side down, and cook for four to five minutes. After that, turn the mushrooms oven and grill them for a further four to five minutes, or until they are soft.

Prepare the avocado, tomato, and lettuce for the burger assembly while the mushrooms are cooking. After the mushrooms are perfectly cooked, take them from the grill and start putting the burgers together.

Top each portobello mushroom with sliced avocado, tomato, and lettuce and place it on a gluten-free hamburger bun or lettuce wrap.

To maintain a low FODMAP and gluten-free meal that is appropriate for individuals with sensitivity to gluten, serve the burgers on lettuce wraps or gluten-free hamburger buns. Serve these burgers with roasted vegetables or a side salad.

Eggplant Parmesan and Vegan Cheese

Serving	Kcal	Carbs	Proteins	Fats	Fiber
4	300	3pg	8g	15g	8g

Prep Time: 30 minutes
Cooking Time: 40 minutes
Total Time: 1 hour 10 minutes

Ingredients

- 1 large eggplant, sliced into 1/4-inch rounds
- 1 cup gluten-free breadcrumbs or almond flour
- 1 teaspoon dried oregano
- 1 teaspoon dried basil
- 1/2 teaspoon garlic powder
- Salt, pepper
- 2 tablespoons olive oil
- 2 cups marinara sauce
- 1 cup vegan mozzarella cheese, shredded
- Fresh basil leaves

Step by Step Preparations

Start by preheating the oven to 400°F (200°C) and line a baking sheet with parchment paper. In a small dish, mix together the gluten-free breadcrumbs or almond flour with dried oregano, dried basil, garlic powder, salt, and pepper.

Dredge each eggplant slice in the breadcrumb mixture, ensuring both sides are uniformly covered. Then, lay the oiled eggplant slices on the prepared baking sheet.

Drizzle olive oil over the coated eggplant slices for extra flavor. Bake the eggplant slices in the preheated oven for 20-25 minutes, or until they become golden brown and soft.

While the eggplant is roasting, reheat the marinara sauce in a small skillet over medium heat until it's cooked through. Once the eggplant slices are done baking, remove them from the oven, but leave the oven on.

Spread a thin layer of marinara sauce on the bottom of a baking dish. Then, put the roasted eggplant slices on top of the sauce.

Sprinkle vegan mozzarella cheese over the eggplant slices, continuing the layers until all the eggplant pieces are used, then concluding with a layer of marinara sauce and vegan cheese on top.

Bake the completed eggplant parmesan in the oven for a further 15 minutes, or until the cheese is melted and bubbling. Before serving, garnish with fresh basil leaves.

You can serve this Eggplant Parmesan as a side dish with grilled chicken or fish, or as a main course with roasted vegetables or salad.

Spinach and Ricotta Stuffed Pasta Shells

Serving	Kcal	Carbs	Proteins	Fats	Fiber
4	350	40g	20g	12g	5g

Prep Time: 20 minutes
Cooking Time: 30 minutes
Total Time: 50 minutes

Ingredients

- 20 jumbo pasta shells
- 2 cups low-fat ricotta cheese
- 1 cup chopped spinach, cooked and drained
- 1/4 cup grated Parmesan cheese
- 1 egg, lightly beaten
- 1/2 teaspoon dried oregano
- 1/2 teaspoon dried basil
- Salt, pepper
- 2 cups tomato sauce
- Fresh basil leaves

Step by Step Preparations

Start by preheating the oven to 375°F (190°C). Lightly oil a 9x13-inch baking dish and lay it aside for later use. Follow the package directions to boil the giant pasta shells until they attain an al dente consistency. Once cooked, drain them and allow them to cool down.

In a spacious mixing basin, add the ricotta cheese, chopped spinach, grated Parmesan cheese, beaten egg, dried oregano, dried basil, salt, and pepper. Ensure vigorous mixing until all ingredients are completely mixed.

Carefully pour the spinach and ricotta mixture into each cooked pasta shell, dividing it equally among them. Arrange the filled shells in the prepared baking dish.

Evenly pour the tomato sauce over the packed shells, ensuring they are thoroughly coated. Cover the baking dish with aluminum foil and bake it in the preheated oven for 20-25 minutes, or until the sauce starts to boil and the shells are cooked through.

Once the first baking time is complete, remove the foil and continue baking for an additional 5 minutes, or until the tops of the shells acquire a light golden tint.

Once completely cooked, remove the dish from the oven and allow the filled shells to cool for a few minutes before serving. Garnish the dish with fresh basil leaves immediately before serving, and eat while hot.

Found in most grocery stores' pasta aisle, jumbo pasta shells are a convenient and adaptable option for stuffing with a variety of fillings. Serve this dish on its own or with a side salad for a complete meal; just make sure to choose a low FODMAP tomato sauce or make your own with fresh tomatoes and herbs.

Vegetable Pad Thai with Tofu

Serving	Kcal	Carbs	Proteins	Fats	Fiber
4	400	45g	15g	20g	5g

Prep Time: 20 minutes
Cooking Time: 15 minutes
Total Time: 35 minutes

Ingredients

- 8 oz rice noodles (Pad Thai noodles)
- 1 block (14 oz) firm tofu, pressed and cubed
- 2 cups bean sprouts
- 1 bell pepper, thinly sliced
- 1 carrot, julienned
- 3 green onions, sliced
- 2 cloves garlic, minced
- 2 tablespoons olive oil
- 2 eggs, lightly beaten
- 1/4 cup roasted peanuts, chopped
- Fresh cilantro
- Lime wedges

Pad Thai Sauce:

- 3 tablespoons low-sodium tamari or soy sauce
- 2 tablespoons rice vinegar
- 1 tablespoon maple syrup or brown sugar
- 1 tablespoon lime juice
- 1 teaspoon grated ginger

- 1 teaspoon sriracha or chili paste

Step by Step Preparations

Commence by cooking the rice noodles according to the directions on the box until they attain an al dente texture. Once cooked, drain them and keep away for later use.

In a small bowl, add all the ingredients for the Pad Thai sauce, whisking them together completely. Set the sauce aside.

In a generous-sized pan or wok, heat 1 tablespoon of olive oil over medium-high heat. Add the cubed tofu and fry until it gets golden brown on both sides, which normally takes approximately 5-6 minutes. Once browned, remove the tofu from the pan and leave it aside for now.

In the same skillet, add the remaining tablespoon of olive oil. Introduce the minced garlic and let it simmer for approximately 1 minute until it emits its delicious scent.

Incorporate the sliced bell pepper and julienned carrot into the skillet. Cook the veggies for 3-4 minutes until they slightly soften. If incorporating eggs, make room in the pan by putting the veggies to one side. Pour the beaten eggs into the designated area and scramble them until thoroughly cooked. Then, combine the eggs with the veggies.

Now, add the cooked rice noodles, bean sprouts, green onions, and the cooked tofu to the pan. Pour the prepared Pad Thai sauce over the mixture, stirring everything together until well incorporated and cooked through.

Once hot, remove the pan from the heat and sprinkle chopped peanuts over the Pad Thai for extra texture and taste. Serve the meal hot, topped with fresh cilantro and lime wedges

For many people with IBS, tofu is an easy-to-digest plant-based source of protein. As for peanuts, they are a good source of protein and healthy fats, but watch portion sizes as they can be high in fat. If you want to cut down on sodium, go for unsalted peanuts. You can also add other vegetables to this Vegetable Pad Thai, like broccoli, cabbage, or snow peas

Vegetarian Sushi Rolls and Carrot

Serving	Kcal	Carbs	Proteins	Fats	Fiber
4 rolls	200	40g	3g	4g	5g

Prep Time: 20 minutes
Cooking Time: 0
Total Time: 20 minutes

Ingredients

- 4 nori seaweed sheets
- 1 cup sushi rice, cooked according to package instructions and seasoned with rice vinegar, sugar, and salt
- 1 avocado, sliced
- 1 cucumber, julienned
- 1 carrot, julienned
- Soy sauce, pickled ginger, wasabi

Step by Step Preparations

Begin by laying a nori seaweed sheet shiny side down on a bamboo sushi mat or a clean kitchen towel.

Spread a layer of sushi rice evenly over the nori sheet, leaving 1 inch of space at the top border. Arrange slices of avocado, julienned cucumber, and julienned carrot in a single layer on the bottom two-thirds of the rice-covered nori sheet.

Starting from the bottom edge closest to you, firmly roll the sushi using the bamboo mat or kitchen towel, using slight pressure as you roll to achieve a secure closure.

Dampen the top edge of the nori sheet slightly with water to seal the roll.
Repeat the procedure with the remaining nori sheets and ingredients.

Once all rolls are constructed, use a sharp knife to slice each roll into 6-8 pieces. Serve the sushi rolls accompanied with soy sauce, pickled ginger, and wasabi on the side.

This recipe is highly customizable; feel free to add or substitute your favorite vegetables or proteins to suit your tastes. Nori seaweed is rich in minerals like iodine and iron, as well as vitamins like vitamin A and C. Sushi rice, when seasoned with rice vinegar, sugar, and salt, provides the perfect sticky texture and mild sweetness that complements the fresh vegetables.

Roasted Vegetable Pizza and Red Onion

Serving	Kcal	Carbs	Proteins	Fats	Fiber
4	300	40g	10g	12g	5g

Prep Time: 15 minutes
Cooking Time: 20 minutes
Total Time: 35 minutes

Ingredients

- 1 pre-made gluten-free or pizza crust
- 1 red bell pepper, thinly sliced
- 1 yellow bell pepper, thinly sliced
- 1 small zucchini, thinly sliced
- 1/2 red onion, thinly sliced
- 1 tablespoon olive oil
- Salt, pepper
- 1 cup marinara sauce
- 1 cup lactose-free or dairy-free cheese, shredded
- Fresh basil leaves

Step by Step Preparations

Preheat the oven to the temperature stated on the pizza crust container. On a baking sheet, place the sliced bell peppers, zucchini, and red onion. Drizzle them with olive oil and season with salt and pepper, achieving a uniform coating.

Roast the seasoned veggies in the preheated oven for 10-15 minutes, until they become soft and have a subtle caramelized texture. Once done, take them from the oven and leave aside.

While the veggies are roasting, evenly distribute marinara sauce over the premade pizza dough. Sprinkle the shredded cheese over the marinara sauce, creating a cheesy foundation.

Top the cheese with the roasted veggies, putting them in a uniform layer. Return the constructed pizza to the oven and bake according to the directions on the pizza crust box, until the crust gets a golden brown tone and the cheese melts and forms bubbles.

Once the pizza is entirely cooked, gently remove it from the oven and allow it to cool slightly before slicing. Before serving, top the pizza with fresh basil leaves for a blast of flavor. Slice the pizza and serve it while still warm.

This pizza is ideal for a quick weeknight dinner or a laid-back get-together with friends. It is made quickly and simply by using a pre-made gluten-free or low FODMAP pizza crust. Look for crusts made with alternative flours like rice flour, almond flour, or tapioca starch. Roasting the vegetables brings out their flavors and adds sweetness to the pizza. Check the ingredient list for high FODMAP ingredients like garlic and onion, and choose a sauce without these additives.

Veggie Wrap with Goat Cheese

Serving	Kcal	Carbs	Proteins	Fats	Fiber
2	350	30g	12g	20g	7g

Prep Time: 20 minutes
Cooking Time: 10 minutes
Total Time: 30 minutes

Ingredients

2 large whole grain or gluten-free tortillas

1 medium zucchini, sliced lengthwise

1 medium yellow squash, sliced lengthwise

1 red bell pepper, sliced into strips

1 yellow bell pepper, sliced into strips

1 tablespoon olive oil

Salt and pepper

2 ounces goat cheese, crumbled

2 tablespoons pesto (store-bought or homemade)

Spinach or arugula leaves, a handful will do just fine.

Step by Step Preparations

Preheat your grill pan or outdoor grill to medium-high heat. Brush olive oil over the zucchini, yellow squash, and bell pepper slices, then season with salt and pepper.

Grill the veggies for 3-4 minutes on each side until they are soft and acquire a little sear. Once done, take them from the grill and put them aside.

Arrange the tortillas on a clean board, then equally distribute 1 tablespoon of pesto over each one. Divide the grilled veggies among the tortillas, laying them in a line along the middle.

Sprinkle crumbled goat cheese over the grilled veggies on each tortilla, followed by a handful of spinach or arugula leaves. Roll up the tortillas firmly, folding in the sides as you go, to make wraps.

For serving, split each wrap in half diagonally. They may be served immediately or wrapped firmly in foil or parchment paper for later

---

These wraps are a great option for lunch or dinner because they're portable and easy to digest. Grilled vegetables are rich in vitamins, minerals, and antioxidants. Grilling also enhances their flavor and gives the wrap a smoky depth.

Quinoa Stuffed Acorn Squash

Serving	Kcal	Carbs	Proteins	Fats	Fiber
4	350	60g	7g	10g	9g

Prep Time: 15 minutes
Cooking Time: 45 minutes
Total Time: 1 hour

Ingredients

- 2 medium acorn squash
- 1 cup quinoa, rinsed
- 2 cups water or vegetable broth
- 1/2 cup dried cranberries
- 1/2 cup pecans, chopped
- 1 tablespoon olive oil
- 1 tablespoon maple syrup
- 1 teaspoon ground cinnamon
- Salt, pepper, fresh parsley

Step by Step Preparations

To start, preheat your oven to 375°F (190°C). Then split the acorn squash in half lengthwise and scrape out the seeds and stringy pulp. Place the squash halves cut-side down on a baking sheet lined with parchment paper.

Bake the squash in the preheated oven for 30-35 minutes, or until they are soft when probed with a fork.

While the squash is baking, prepare the quinoa. In a medium saucepan, bring water or vegetable broth to a boil. Add the quinoa, then decrease the heat to low, cover, and simmer for approximately 15 minutes, or until the quinoa is cooked and the water is absorbed. Once done, take it from the fire and let it cool slightly.

In a large mixing bowl, combine the cooked quinoa, dried cranberries, chopped nuts, olive oil, maple syrup, ground cinnamon, salt, and pepper. Stir the mixture until everything is fully blended.

Once the squash halves are cooked, take them from the oven and gently turn them over. Fill each squash half with the quinoa mixture, maintaining a uniform distribution.

Return the filled squash to the oven and bake for a further 10-15 minutes, or until the stuffing is cooked through and the tops are gently brown. Before serving, sprinkle with fresh parsley to provide a finishing touch.

You can eat this stuffed acorn squash as a filling side dish or as a main course with grilled chicken or fish.

GLUTEN-FREE AND DAIRY-FREE OPTIONS

(Choose Low FODMAP Ingredients when necessary; The list in Appendices will guide you).

Grilled Salmon with Steamed Vegetables

Serving	Kcal	Carbs	Proteins	Fats	Fiber
4	400	25g	30g	20g	5g

Prep Time: 15 minutes
Cooking Time: 15 minutes
Total Time: 30 minutes

Ingredients

4 salmon filets (about 6 oz each), skin removed

2 cups carrots, broccoli, and bell peppers, cut into bite-sized pieces

1 cup quinoa, rinsed

2 cups water or vegetable broth

2 tablespoons olive oil

Salt, pepper, fresh lemon wedges, fresh herbs

Step by Step Preparations

Preheat your grill to medium-high heat, ensuring it's ready for grilling. Meanwhile, season the salmon filets with salt, pepper, and a dab of olive oil to enhance their taste.

Once the grill is hot, gently lay the seasoned salmon filets on it and cook them for 4-5 minutes each side. Keep an eye on them and ensure they are cooked through and readily flake with a fork. Once done, take the salmon from the grill and lay it aside shortly.

While the salmon is cooking, shift your focus to making the quinoa. In a medium saucepan, bring either water or vegetable broth to a boil. Add the rinsed quinoa, then decrease the heat to low, cover, and let it simmer for approximately 15 minutes, enabling the quinoa to cook properly and absorb the liquid. Once cooked, fluff the quinoa with a fork and leave it aside.

In a separate pot fitted with a steamer basket, bring approximately an inch of water to a boil. Add the mixed veggies to the steamer basket, cover it, and let the vegetables cook for 5-7 minutes, or until they attain a tender-crisp texture.

To create the meal, divide the cooked quinoa across plates, forming a foundation. Top the quinoa with the steamed veggies, dividing them evenly. Finally, lay a cooked salmon filet on each platter. For a final touch, garnish the meal with fresh lemon wedges and herbs to add brightness and flavor.

This dish can be eaten for lunch or dinner and is well-balanced and nutritious, with a good combination of protein, carbs, and healthy fats.

Quinoa Salad with Roasted Vegetables

Serving	Kcal	Carbs	Proteins	Fats	Fiber
4	300	30g	8g	18g	6g

Prep Time: 15 minutes
Cooking Time: 25 minutes
Total Time: 40 minutes

Ingredients

1 cup quinoa, rinsed

2 cups water or vegetable broth

2 cups bell peppers, zucchini, cherry tomatoes, diced

2 tablespoons olive oil

Salt and pepper

1/4 cup fresh parsley, chopped

1/4 cup fresh basil leaves, chopped

Lemon-Tahini Dressing:

1/4 cup tahini

2 tablespoons lemon juice

2 tablespoons water

1 clove garlic, minced

Salt and pepper

Step by Step Preparations

Start by preheating the oven to 400°F (200°C) and lining a baking sheet with parchment paper for easy cleanup.

In a medium saucepan, bring water or vegetable broth to a boil. Add the quinoa, then reduce the heat to low, cover, and let it simmer for about 15 minutes until the quinoa is cooked and the liquid is absorbed. Once done, remove it from the heat and allow it to cool slightly.

While the quinoa is cooking, spread the diced vegetables evenly on the prepared baking sheet. Drizzle them with olive oil and season with salt and pepper, ensuring they're coated evenly.

Roast the seasoned vegetables in the preheated oven for 20-25 minutes, or until they're tender and develop a slight caramelization, remembering to stir them halfway through cooking for even browning.

In a spacious mixing bowl, combine the cooked quinoa, roasted vegetables, chopped parsley, and basil. In a separate small bowl, whisk together the tahini, lemon juice, water, minced garlic, salt, and pepper until a smooth, creamy dressing forms.

Pour the lemon-tahini dressing over the quinoa and vegetable mixture, gently tossing until everything is thoroughly coated. Lastly, taste the dish and adjust the seasoning

---

This salad can be enjoyed as a light lunch or dinner option, or as a side dish alongside grilled chicken or fish. Tahini is a sesame seed that's a good source of healthy fats and adds richness without dairy. If you are sensitive to FODMAPs or have a garlic intolerance, omit the garlic.

Chicken, Vegetable Stir-Fry and Brown Rice

Serving	Kcal	Carbs	Proteins	Fats	Fiber
4	350	35g	25g	12g	6g

Prep Time: 15 minutes
Cooking Time: 15 minutes
Total Time: 30 minutes

Ingredients

- 2 boneless, skinless chicken breasts, thinly sliced
- 2 cups bell peppers, broccoli, snap peas, sliced or chopped
- 2 cloves garlic, minced
- 1 tablespoon ginger, minced
- 3 tablespoons tamari sauce
- 2 tablespoons olive oil
- 4 cups cooked brown rice
- Salt, pepper, sesame seeds, sliced green onions

Step by Step Preparations

Begin by heating 1 tablespoon of olive oil in a large skillet or wok over medium-high heat. Introduce the sliced chicken breasts and heat them until they attain a browned, cooked-through consistency, 5-6 minutes. Once done, take the chicken from the pan and put it aside shortly.

In the same skillet, combine the remaining tablespoon of olive oil. Add the minced garlic and ginger, letting them simmer for approximately 1 minute until they exude a fragrant scent.

Next, add the mixed veggies to the pan and stir-fry them for 3-4 minutes, until they achieve a crisp-tender stage.

Reintroduce the cooked chicken to the skillet. Pour the tamari sauce over the chicken and veggies, ensuring uniform covering by tossing everything together. Allow the mixture to simmer for another 1-2 minutes to heat thoroughly.

Season the meal with salt and pepper according to taste preferences. Serve the fragrant chicken and vegetable stir-fry over cooked brown rice. Garnish the meal with sesame seeds and chopped green onions for an extra touch of taste

---

Brown rice is a whole grain rich in fiber, which helps with digestion and helps regulate bowel movements. It also provides sustained energy and helps keep you feeling full and satisfied. Chicken provides lean protein, which is easy to digest and can help maintain muscle mass and energy levels.

Baked Chicken Breast and Sautéed Spinach

Serving	Kcal	Carbs	Proteins	Fats	Fiber
4	350	30g	30g	12g	6g

Prep Time: 15 minutes
Cooking Time: 40 minutes
Total Time: 55 minutes

Ingredients

4 boneless, skinless chicken breasts

2 large sweet potatoes, peeled and diced

4 cups fresh spinach leaves

2 tablespoons olive oil, divided

2 cloves garlic, minced

Salt, pepper, fresh chopped parsley

Step by Step Preparations

To begin, preheat your oven to 400°F (200°C). In a big saucepan, immerse the chopped sweet potatoes in water. Bring the saucepan to a boil and allow the sweet potatoes simmer for 15-20 minutes until they are soft when poked with a fork.

While the sweet potatoes are cooking, season both sides of the chicken breasts with salt and pepper.

In a large skillet over medium-high heat, warm 1 tablespoon of olive oil. Add the seasoned chicken breasts and fry them for 3-4 minutes on each side until they attain a golden brown color.

Transfer the browned chicken breasts to a baking dish and set them in the preheated oven. Let them bake for 20-25 minutes until they are thoroughly done and no longer pink in the middle.

Meanwhile, in the same pan used for frying the chicken, heat the remaining 1 tablespoon of olive oil over medium heat. Add the minced garlic and heat it for 1-2 minutes until it turns aromatic.

Incorporate the fresh spinach into the pan and sauté it for 3-4 minutes until it wilts. Season the spinach with salt and pepper according to your taste.

Once the sweet potatoes are soft, drain them and return them to the saucepan. Mash the sweet potatoes with a potato masher until they attain a smooth and creamy consistency. Season the mashed sweet potatoes with salt and pepper to taste. Serve with the creamy sweet potato mash and sautéed spinach

---

Without adding dairy or too much saturated fat, olive oil gives the chicken and vegetables a rich flavor. It is a good source of monounsaturated fats.

Shrimp and Avocado Salad

Serving	Kcal	Carbs	Proteins	Fats	Fiber
4	300	15g	20g	20g	8g

Prep Time: 15 minutes
Cooking Time: 5 minutes
Total Time: 20 minutes

Ingredients

- 1 pound shrimp, peeled and deveined
- 2 avocados, diced
- 6 cups spinach, arugula, and lettuce
- 1/4 cup cherry tomatoes, halved
- 1/4 cup cucumber, sliced
- 1/4 cup red onion, thinly sliced
- 1/4 cup balsamic vinegar
- 2 tablespoons olive oil
- 1 teaspoon Dijon mustard
- Salt, pepper, fresh basil leaves

Step by Step Preparations

In a big pan, heat a drizzle of olive oil over medium-high heat. Introduce the shrimp and fry them for 2-3 minutes on each side till they become pink and cook through.

Once done, remove the pan from heat and allow the shrimp to cool slightly. Meanwhile, in a separate bowl, mix together the balsamic vinegar, olive oil, Dijon mustard, salt, and pepper to create the vinaigrette.

In a spacious salad bowl, add the mixed greens, diced avocado, cherry tomatoes, sliced cucumber, and red onion. Add the cooked shrimp to the salad dish.

Drizzle the prepared balsamic vinaigrette over the salad and carefully mix to ensure all components are well covered. Taste the salad and adjust spice

---

Shrimp is an easily digestible, low-FODMAP protein source that is appropriate for people with IBS. It is also a good source of omega-3 fatty acids, which have the potential to lower inflammation and promote gut health.

Turkey Meatballs with Spaghetti Squash

Serving	Kcal	Carbs	Proteins	Fats	Fiber
4	350	20g	30g	15g	5g

Prep Time: 20 minutes
Cooking Time: 1 hour
Total Time: 1 hour 20 minutes

Ingredients

- 1 medium spaghetti squash
- 1 lb ground turkey
- 1/4 cup gluten-free breadcrumbs
- 1 egg
- 1/4 cup grated Parmesan cheese
- 1 teaspoon dried oregano
- 1 teaspoon dried basil
- 1/2 teaspoon garlic powder
- Salt and pepper
- 2 cups marinara sauce
- Fresh parsley

Step by Step Preparations

Start by preheating the oven to 400°F (200°C). Proceed to split the spaghetti squash lengthwise and remove the seeds. Place the squash halves cut side down on a baking sheet lined with parchment paper.

Bake them for 40-45 minutes, or until the squash assumes a soft consistency and can be readily punctured with a fork.

While the squash is baking, make the turkey meatballs. In a large mixing bowl, combine the ground turkey, gluten-free breadcrumbs, egg, Parmesan cheese, dried oregano, dried basil, garlic powder, salt, and pepper. Mix the ingredients until they are fully blended.

Shape the turkey mixture into meatballs, aiming for sizes approximately 1-2 inches in diameter, and lay them on a baking sheet lined with parchment paper. Bake the meatballs in the preheated oven for 20-25 minutes, or until they are thoroughly cooked through and acquire a lightly browned surface.

Meanwhile, cook the marinara sauce in a skillet over medium heat until it is heated through. Once the spaghetti squash is done, use a fork to scrape the meat into strands. Divide the strands of squash among serving dishes. Top the spaghetti squash with marinara sauce and the newly cooked turkey meatballs.

Ground turkey is a lean source of protein that is easier to digest than red meat, making it a suitable option for those with IBS. Gluten-free breadcrumbs are used to bind the turkey meatballs together without triggering symptoms in individuals with gluten sensitivities. Parmesan cheese adds flavor to the meatballs but can be omitted if dairy is a problem. Spaghetti squash is a low-FODMAP alternative to traditional pasta, making it suitable for individuals with IBS who are sensitive to wheat and gluten.

Lentil Soup with Carrots and Kale

Serving	Kcal	Carbs	Proteins	Fats	Fiber
4	250	35g	12g	7g	12g

Prep Time: 15 minutes
Cooking Time: 30 minutes
Total Time: 45 minutes

Ingredients

- 1 cup dry green or brown lentils, rinsed and drained
- 4 cups vegetable broth
- 2 carrots, diced
- 2 stalks celery, diced
- 2 cups kale, chopped
- 2 tablespoons olive oil
- 2 cloves garlic, minced
- 1 teaspoon dried thyme
- Salt, pepper, fresh lemon wedges

Step by Step Preparations

Begin by heating olive oil in a large saucepan over medium heat. Incorporate the chopped carrots and celery, letting them simmer for 5 minutes until they soften somewhat.

Introduce minced garlic to the saucepan, simmering for a further 1-2 minutes until its scent becomes aromatic. Proceed to whisk in rinsed lentils, vegetable broth, dried thyme, salt, and pepper. Bring the soup to a boil. Once boiling, decrease the heat to low, cover the pot, and let the soup simmer for approximately 20-25 minutes, or until the lentils achieve a soft consistency.

Add chopped kale to the saucepan and stir until it wilts, which normally takes approximately 2-3 minutes. Taste the soup and adjust the flavor by adding additional salt and pepper

---

You can have this soup by itself as a satisfying meal or with a slice of low-FODMAPS bread for something a little heavier.

Grilled Steak with Roasted Brussels Sprouts

Serving	Kcal	Carbs	Proteins	Fats	Fiber
4	500	25g	35g	30g	5g

Prep Time: 15 minutes
Marinating Time: 30 minutes
Cooking Time: 30 minutes
Total Time: 1 hour 15 minutes

For the Grilled Steak

- 4 boneless beef steaks, sirloin or ribeye, about 6 oz each
- 2 tablespoons olive oil
- 2 cloves garlic, minced
- 1 tablespoon fresh rosemary, chopped
- Salt and pepper

For the Roasted Brussels Sprouts

- 1 lb Brussels sprouts, trimmed and halved
- 2 tablespoons olive oil
- 1 teaspoon smoked paprika
- Salt and pepper

For the Wild Rice

- 1 cup wild rice
- 2 cups water vegetable broth
- Salt

Step by Step Preparations

For the Grilled Steak

Start by mixing together the olive oil, minced garlic, chopped rosemary, salt, and pepper in a small bowl.

Place the steaks in a shallow dish or resealable plastic bag, then pour the marinade over them, ensuring each steak is well covered. Let the steaks marinate in the refrigerator for at least 30 minutes, or up to 4 hours for optimum flavor absorption.

Preheat the grill to medium-high heat. Remove the steaks from the marinade, discarding any excess. Grill the steaks for 4-6 minutes each side, or until they achieve your preferred amount of doneness. Once done, remove the steaks from the grill and allow them to rest for a few minutes before serving.

For the Roasted Brussels Sprouts

Start by preheating the oven to 400°F (200°C) and line a baking sheet with parchment paper. In a large bowl, mix the Brussels sprouts with olive oil, smoked paprika, salt, and pepper, tossing until they are uniformly coated.

Spread the seasoned Brussels sprouts out in a single layer on the prepared baking sheet. Roast the Brussels sprouts in the preheated oven for 20-25 minutes, or until they become soft and have a caramelized surface, remembering to stir halfway during the cooking procedure.

For the Wild Rice

In a medium pot, join the wild rice, water or vegetable broth, and salt. Initiate by bringing the mixture to a boil, then decrease the heat to a slow simmer. Cover the pot and let it boil for 40-45 minutes until the rice gets a soft texture and absorbs the liquid totally.

Once done, remove the pot from heat and let it remain, covered, for an additional 5 minutes to enable the flavors to settle. After the resting time, lightly fluff the rice with a fork before serving.

Serve with a side of low-FODMAP sauce or seasoning of your choice.

Chickpea and Basmati Rice

Serving	Kcal	Carbs	Proteins	Fats	Fiber
4	450	60g	12g	20g	10g

Prep Time: 15 minutes
Cooking Time: 30 minutes
Total Time: 45 minutes

For the Curry

- 1 can (15 oz) chickpeas, drained and rinsed
- 1 can (14 oz) coconut milk
- 2 cups bell peppers, zucchini, and green beans, diced
- 1 onion, finely chopped
- 2 cloves garlic, minced
- 1 tablespoon ginger, minced
- 2 tablespoons curry powder
- 1 teaspoon ground cumin
- 1 teaspoon ground coriander
- 1/2 teaspoon turmeric powder
- 1 tablespoon olive oil
- Salt, pepper, fresh cilantro

For the Basmati Rice

- 1 cup basmati rice
- 2 cups water
- Pinch of salt

Step by Step Preparations

For the Curry

In a large sized pan or pot, warm up the olive oil over medium heat. Introduce the chopped onion and simmer until it becomes transparent, often about 3-4 minutes.

Incorporate the minced garlic and ginger into the pan, letting them simmer for a further 1-2 minutes until they emit their delicious smell.

Next, whisk in the curry powder, powdered cumin, ground coriander, and turmeric powder. Continuously whisk the mixture for approximately 1 minute until the spices become roasted and give an attractive perfume.

Add the mixed veggies to the pan and heat them for 5 minutes, allowing them to soften slightly. Pour in the coconut milk, ensuring it combines well with the other ingredients. Bring the mixture to a medium simmer.

Introduce the chickpeas to the pan, ensuring they are properly covered with the coconut milk and spices. Let the curry simmer for a further 10-15 minutes, stirring regularly, until the veggies attain a tender consistency and the flavors melt together harmoniously. Finally, season the curry with salt and pepper

For the Basmati Rice

Start by washing the basmati rice under cold water until the water runs clear, thereby eliminating any extra starch. In a medium-sized saucepan, mix the washed rice, water, and a bit of salt. Bring the mixture to a boil over high heat.

Once the mixture comes to a boil, decrease the heat to low, cover the pot, and let it simmer for 15-20 minutes, or until the rice is soft and has absorbed all the water.

After simmering, remove the pot from the heat and let it remain, covered, for an additional 5 minutes to enable the rice to steam and fluff up. Finally, fluff the rice with a fork before serving to produce a light and fluffy texture.

With its mild flavor and fluffy texture, basmati rice is an ideal side dish for curries and is a low FODMAP grain that most people with IBS can tolerate.

Vegetable Stir-Fry with Broccoli

Serving	Kcal	Carbs	Proteins	Fats	Fiber
4	350	40g	15g	15g	7g

Prep Time: 15 minutes
Cooking Time: 20 minutes
Total Time: 35 minutes

Ingredients

- 1 cup quinoa, rinsed
- 2 cups water or vegetable broth
- 1 block (14 oz) extra-firm tofu, pressed and cubed
- 2 cups broccoli florets
- 1 bell pepper, sliced
- 1 carrot, thinly sliced
- 2 tablespoons low-sodium soy sauce or tamari
- 1 tablespoon rice vinegar
- 1 tablespoon maple syrup or other sweetener
- 1 teaspoon grated ginger
- 2 cloves garlic, minced
- 2 tablespoons olive oil or sesame oil
- Salt, pepper, sesame seeds, sliced green onions

Step by Step Preparations

Begin by bringing water or vegetable broth to a boil in a medium pot. Once boiling, add the quinoa, then decrease the heat to low, cover, and allow it to simmer for 15 minutes or until the quinoa is cooked and the water is totally absorbed.

Afterward, remove the pot from the heat and let it remain covered for an additional 5 minutes before fluffing the quinoa with a fork.

In a small bowl, add low-sodium soy sauce, rice vinegar, maple syrup, grated ginger, and chopped garlic, stirring them together to produce the stir-fry sauce. Set this mixture aside.

Heat 1 tablespoon of olive oil or sesame oil in a large pan or wok over medium-high heat. Add the cubed tofu and cook for 5-7 minutes, stirring regularly, until it acquires a golden brown color on both sides. Once cooked, remove the tofu from the pan and keep it away for later use.

In the same skillet, add the remaining tablespoon of oil. Introduce the sliced bell peppers and carrots, cooking them for 3-4 minutes until they begin to soften somewhat.

Next, add the broccoli florets to the pan and simmer for an additional 2-3 minutes, ensuring the veggies attain a tender-crisp texture.

Reintroduce the cooked tofu to the pan, then pour the prepared stir-fry sauce over the tofu and veggies. Stir everything up well to evenly coat the items in the sauce. Allow the mixture to simmer for another 2-3 minutes until cooked through.

Taste the stir-fry and adjust the seasoning with salt and pepper if required. Finally, serve the vegetable stir-fry over the cooked quinoa, garnishing it with sesame seeds and sliced green onions for extra taste

---

You can alter this dish by adding your preferred vegetables or protein sources.

Gluten-Free Pasta with Tomato Basil Sauce

Serving	Kcal	Carbs	Proteins	Fats	Fiber
4	400	45g	25g	12g	5g

Prep Time: 15 minutes
Cooking Time: 25 minutes
Total Time: 40 minutes

Ingredients

- 8 ounces brown rice or quinoa pasta
- 2 boneless, skinless chicken breasts
- 2 cups tomato basil pasta sauce
- 1 tablespoon olive oil
- 2 cloves garlic, minced
- Salt, pepper, fresh basil leaves, grated Parmesan cheese

Step by Step Preparations

Commence by cooking the gluten-free pasta following the directions on the box until it achieves an al dente texture. Drain the pasta and keep it aside. Preheat a grill or grill pan over medium-high heat. Season the chicken breasts with salt and pepper.

Grill the seasoned chicken breasts for 6-7 minutes each side, ensuring they are well done and no longer pink in the middle. Once done, take the chicken from the grill and allow it to rest for a few minutes before slicing.

While the chicken is cooking, heat the olive oil in a large pan over medium heat. If using minced garlic, add it to the pan and heat for 1-2 minutes until it gets fragrant. Pour the tomato basil pasta sauce into the pan and reheat it completely.

Introduce the cooked gluten-free spaghetti to the pan holding the tomato basil sauce. Toss the spaghetti carefully to ensure it is properly covered with the sauce.

Serve the spaghetti, liberally covered with sliced grilled chicken breast. For a final touch, sprinkle the meal with fresh basil leaves and grated Parmesan cheese

This dish can be served as a main course for lunch or dinner; avoid using strong marinades or spices that could cause symptoms.

Turkey and Vegetable Chili

Serving	Kcal	Carbs	Proteins	Fats	Fiber
4	300	25g	25g	10g	8g

Prep Time: 15 minutes
Cooking Time: 30 minutes
Total Time: 45 minutes

Ingredients

- 1 pound ground turkey
- 1 can (15 oz) kidney beans, drained and rinsed
- 1 can (14.5 oz) crushed tomatoes
- 1 onion, diced
- 2 cloves garlic, minced
- 1 bell pepper, diced
- 1 zucchini, diced
- 1 tablespoon olive oil
- 1 tablespoon chili powder
- 1 teaspoon ground cumin
- 1/2 teaspoon paprika
- Salt, pepper, fresh cilantro, lime wedges

Step by Step Preparations

In a large sized saucepan or Dutch oven, preheat the olive oil over medium heat. Sauté the chopped onion until it softens, normally about 3-4 minutes.

Introduce the minced garlic to the saucepan, letting it simmer for a further 1-2 minutes until its scent becomes aromatic. Incorporate the ground turkey into the saucepan, breaking it up with a spoon as it browns and cooks completely, generally taking 5-7 minutes.

Add the chopped bell pepper and zucchini to the saucepan, simmering them for another 3-4 minutes until they slightly soften. Sprinkle the chili powder, ground cumin, paprika, salt, and pepper over the meat and veggies, stirring well to ensure they are uniformly covered with the spices.

Pour in the smashed tomatoes and kidney beans, stirring well to mix all the ingredients. Bring the chili to a medium simmer.

Allow the chili to boil for 15-20 minutes, stirring regularly, until the flavors merge together, and the chili achieves your ideal thickness. Taste the chili and adjust the spice before serving.

For added taste and texture, this chili can also be served with toppings like shredded cheese, diced red onion, or avocado slices.

Baked Cod and Quinoa Pilaf

Serving	Kcal	Carbs	Proteins	Fats	Fiber
4	350	30g	30g	12g	6g

Prep Time: 15 minutes
Cooking Time: 25 minutes
Total Time: 40 minutes

For the Baked Cod

- 4 cod filets (about 6 oz each)
- 2 tablespoons olive oil
- 2 cloves garlic, minced
- 1 tablespoon lemon juice
- Salt and pepper

For the Roasted Asparagus

- 1 bunch asparagus, trimmed
- 1 tablespoon olive oil
- Salt and pepper

For the Quinoa Pilaf

- 1 cup quinoa, rinsed
- 2 cups vegetable broth
- 1 tablespoon olive oil
- 1/4 cup diced bell pepper
- 1/4 cup diced carrot
- 1/4 cup diced zucchini
- 2 tablespoons chopped fresh parsley
- Salt and pepper

Step by Step Preparations

For the Baked Cod

Preheat your oven to 375°F (190°C) to ensure it's ready for baking. In a small bowl, add the olive oil, minced garlic, lemon juice, salt, and pepper, stirring them together completely.

Arrange the cod filets on a baking pan lined with either parchment paper or aluminum foil. Using a brush, evenly coat the cod filets with the olive oil mixture. Place the baking sheet with the cod in the preheated oven and bake for 12-15 minutes, or until the fish is thoroughly cooked and readily flakes with a fork.

Now, for the Roasted Asparagus: While the cod is baking, prepare another baking sheet and lay the trimmed asparagus stalks on it. Drizzle the asparagus spears with olive oil and season them with salt & pepper to taste. Transfer the baking sheet with the asparagus to the preheated oven and roast for around 10-12 minutes, ensuring they stay soft but crisp.

For the Quinoa Pilaf

Start by heating 1 tablespoon of olive oil in a medium saucepan over medium heat.
Introduce the chopped bell pepper, carrot, and zucchini to the pot, allowing them to fry for 3-4 minutes until they slightly soften.

Add the washed quinoa to the pot, stirring to ensure it's equally covered with the veggies and oil. Proceed by adding in the low FODMAP vegetable broth, bringing it to a boil.

Once boiling, decrease the heat to low, cover the pot, and allow it to simmer for 15 minutes, or until the quinoa is completely cooked and the liquid is absorbed. Using a fork, fluff the quinoa pilaf and then toss in the chopped parsley. Season with salt and pepper

Cod is a mild-flavored, low-fat fish that is easy to digest and can be a good option for people with IBS. You can change up the vegetables in the quinoa pilaf according to what's in season. Diced cucumber, cherry tomatoes, or spinach are some other options.

Eggplant and Zucchini Lasagna

Serving	Kcal	Carbs	Proteins	Fats	Fiber
6	250	20g	8g	15g	5g

Prep Time: 20 minutes
Cooking Time: 45 minutes
Total Time: 1 hour 5 minutes

Ingredients

- 1 large eggplant, sliced lengthwise into 1/4-inch thick slices
- 2 medium zucchinis, sliced lengthwise into 1/4-inch thick slices
- 2 cups almond or cashew cheese
- 2 cups tomato sauce
- 2 tablespoons olive oil
- 2 cloves garlic, minced
- 1 teaspoon dried oregano
- 1 teaspoon dried basil
- Salt and pepper

Step by Step Preparations

Start by preheating your oven to 375°F (190°C) and liberally greasing a 9x13 inch baking dish with olive oil. Arrange the eggplant and zucchini slices on a parchment paper-lined baking sheet.

Drizzle them with olive oil and sprinkle over minced garlic, dried oregano, dried basil, salt, and pepper. Toss lightly to ensure uniform coating.

Roast the seasoned eggplant and zucchini slices in the preheated oven for 15-20 minutes, or until they become soft. Once done, take them from the oven and allow them to cool slightly.

In the prepared baking dish, apply a thin layer of tomato sauce on the bottom. Arrange half of the roasted eggplant and zucchini pieces on top of the sauce.

Sprinkle half of the dairy-free cheese over the veggie layer. Repeat the stacking technique with another layer of tomato sauce, the remaining roasted veggies, and the remaining dairy-free cheese.

Cover the baking dish with aluminum foil and bake it in the preheated oven for 25-30 minutes, or until the cheese is melted and bubbling.

Remove the foil and bake for a further 5-10 minutes, or until the top gets a gently golden brown tint. Allow the lasagna to cool for a few minutes before slicing and serving.

To make this lasagna more nutrient-dense and flavorful, try layering on some spinach or mushrooms. You can also add other vegetables or herbs.

Spinach with Gluten-Free Toast

Serving	Kcal	Carbs	Proteins	Fats	Fiber
1	250	10g	15g	17g	3g

Prep Time: 10 minutes
Cooking Time: 10 minutes
Total Time: 20 minutes

Ingredients

- 2 large eggs
- 1 cup fresh spinach leaves
- 1/2 cup sliced mushrooms
- 1 tablespoon olive oil
- Salt and pepper
- 1 slice gluten-free bread
- Cooking spray

Step by Step Preparations

In a small bowl, whisk the eggs using a fork until fully blended. Season with salt. In a non-stick skillet over medium heat, preheat the olive oil. Add the sliced mushrooms and sauté them for 2-3 minutes until they begin to soften.

Introduce the fresh spinach leaves to the pan and heat for an additional 1-2 minutes until they wilt. Pour the beaten eggs over the mushrooms and spinach in the skillet, gently rotating the pan to achieve uniform dispersion of the eggs.

Allow the omelet to cook undisturbed for 3-4 minutes, frequently raising the sides with a spatula to allow the raw egg flow below, until the bottom is set and the top is slightly runny.

With care, fold the omelet in half using the spatula and continue cooking for another 1-2 minutes until the eggs are completely cooked and the omelet attains a golden brown appearance on both sides.

While the omelet is cooking, toast the gluten-free bread until it gets a golden brown hue. You may do this with a toaster or by toasting it in a pan with a little coating of cooking spray or olive oil over medium heat. Serve the freshly made omelet hot with the toasted gluten-free bread.

Savor this omelet for brunch or breakfast, or simply as a quick and simple dinner at any time of day.

Tofu and Vegetable Pad Thai

Serving	Kcal	Carbs	Proteins	Fats	Fiber
4	400	50g	15g	18g	7g

Prep Time: 20 minutes
Cooking Time: 20 minutes
Total Time: 40 minutes

Ingredients

- 8 oz rice noodles (pad Thai noodles)
- 1 block (14 oz) firm tofu, pressed and cubed
- 2 cups bell peppers, carrots, and broccoli, thinly sliced
- 2 cups bean sprouts
- 3 green onions, chopped
- 3 cloves garlic, minced
- 2 eggs, beaten
- 1/4 cup peanuts, chopped
- 2 tablespoons vegetable oil
- 2 tablespoons soy sauce or tamari
- 2 tablespoons tamarind paste or rice vinegar
- 1 tablespoon brown sugar
- 1 tablespoon lime juice
- 1 teaspoon chili flakes
- Fresh cilantro, lime wedges

Step by Step Preparations

Begin by cooking the rice noodles as per the package directions until they attain an al dente texture. Once done, drain them and keep them away for later use.

In a small bowl, mix together the soy sauce or tamari, tamarind paste or rice vinegar, brown sugar, lime juice, and chili flakes. Set this sauce mixture aside for now.

In a large skillet or wok, heat 1 tablespoon of vegetable oil over medium-high heat. Add the cubed tofu and fry until they attain a golden brown tone on both sides, 5-7 minutes. Once cooked, remove the tofu from the pan and put it aside.

In the same skillet, add the remaining tablespoon of vegetable oil. Introduce the minced garlic and heat it for around 1 minute until it emits its delicious scent.

Next, add the sliced mixed veggies to the pan and sauté them for 3-5 minutes until they attain a tender-crisp consistency. Push the cooked veggies to one side of the pan and pour the beaten eggs into the vacant side. Scramble the eggs until they are totally cooked, then combine them with the veggies.

Now, add the cooked rice noodles, cooked tofu, bean sprouts, chopped green onions, and the prepared sauce to the pan. Toss everything together until all ingredients are completely blended and cooked through, which should take around 2-3 minutes.

Once everything is cooked thoroughly, remove the pan from the heat source and serve the wonderful stir-fried noodles immediately.

Although they add flavor and crunch to the Pad Thai, peanuts can be left out if you have a nut allergy or are sensitive to them.

Vegan Buddha Bowl and Tahini Sauce

Serving	Kcal	Carbs	Proteins	Fats	Fiber
4	450	55g	15g	20g	12g

Prep Time: 15 minutes
Cooking Time: 30 minutes
Total Time: 45 minutes

For the Roasted Vegetables and Chickpeas

- 2 cups sweet potatoes, broccoli, and cauliflower, diced
- 1 can (15 oz) chickpeas, drained and rinsed
- 2 tablespoons olive oil
- 1 teaspoon ground cumin
- 1 teaspoon paprika
- Salt and pepper

For the Tahini Sauce

- 1/4 cup tahini
- 2 tablespoons lemon juice
- 2 tablespoons water
- 1 clove garlic, minced, Salt

For Assembly

- 4 cups cooked quinoa or brown rice
- Fresh spinach

Step by Step Preparations

Start by preheating the oven to 400°F (200°C). In a wide bowl, add the diced veggies, chickpeas, olive oil, ground cumin, paprika, salt, and pepper, ensuring all components are fully covered.

Spread the seasoned veggies and chickpeas equally on a baking sheet lined with parchment paper. Roast them in the preheated oven for 25-30 minutes, or until the veggies attain softness and the chickpeas become crispy, remembering to stir halfway through.

While the veggies and chickpeas are roasting, make the tahini sauce. In a small bowl, mix together the tahini, lemon juice, water, chopped garlic, and salt until a smooth, creamy consistency is produced. Adjust the thickness of the sauce with extra water if required.

To create the Buddha bowls, spread the cooked quinoa or brown rice equally among four bowls. Top each dish with the roasted veggies and chickpeas.

Drizzle the tahini sauce liberally over each bowl. Complete the Buddha bowls with a dish of fresh spinach or mixed greens.

Quinoa, or brown rice, provides additional protein and complex carbohydrates, making it a wholesome and satisfying base for Buddha bowls.

Roasted Vegetable Salad and Balsamic Glaze

Serving	Kcal	Carbs	Proteins	Fats	Fiber
4	200	15g	3g	15g	7g

Prep Time: 15 minutes
Cooking Time: 25 minutes
Total Time: 40 minutes

Ingredients

- 4 cups spinach, arugula, and romaine
- 1 medium zucchini, sliced
- 1 medium yellow squash, sliced
- 1 red bell pepper, sliced
- 1 yellow bell pepper, sliced
- 1 red onion, sliced
- 1 avocado, diced
- 2 tablespoons olive oil
- Salt and pepper
- Balsamic glaze

Step by Step Preparations

Start by preheating your oven to 400°F (200°C). Arrange the sliced zucchini, yellow squash, red bell pepper, yellow bell pepper, and red onion on a generously sized baking sheet. Drizzle them with olive oil and season with salt and pepper, ensuring each veggie is well covered.

Place the seasoned veggies in the preheated oven and roast them for 20-25 minutes, or until they attain softness and a mild caramelized look, remembering to toss halfway during the cooking procedure.

While the veggies are roasting, prepare the mixed greens by thoroughly washing and drying them. Place the greens in a wide salad dish.

Once the roasted veggies are finished, take them from the oven and allow them to cool somewhat. Add the roasted veggies to the dish of mixed greens, then liberally top with cubed avocado.

Just before serving, sprinkle balsamic glaze over the salad, ensuring it covers the components evenly. Gently mix the salad to incorporate, ensuring all components are uniformly covered balsamic glaze.

Look for a balsamic glaze that doesn't contain any high-FODMAP ingredients or added sugars.

Turkey and Gluten-Free Tortilla

Serving	Kcal	Carbs	Proteins	Fats	Fiber
1 wrap	300	25g	20g	15g	6g

Prep Time: 10 minutes
Cooking Time: 0 min.
Total Time: 10 minutes

Ingredients

1 gluten-free tortilla

3 slices of deli turkey breast

1/2 avocado, sliced

2-3 lettuce leaves

1 small tomato, sliced

1 tablespoon hummus or mayonnaise

Salt and pepper

Step by Step Preparations

Place the gluten-free tortilla flat on a clean surface. Evenly spread hummus or low-FODMAP mayonnaise over the tortilla, careful to leave a little border around the edges.

Arrange deli turkey breast pieces, avocado slices, lettuce leaves, and tomato slices equally on top of the tortilla, dispersing them throughout the surface. Season the filling with salt and pepper to taste. Starting from one end, firmly wrap up the tortilla to surround the contents. Slice the wrap diagonally in half for better handling.

For those with IBS, this wrap is a quick and simple lunch, dinner, or on-the-go snack option.

Quinoa Stuffed Bell Peppers and Salsa

Serving	Kcal	Carbs	Proteins	Fats	Fiber
4	300	55g	10g	4g	12g

Prep Time: 20 minutes
Cooking Time: 35 minutes
Total Time: 55 minutes

Ingredients

- 4 large bell peppers, halved and seeds removed
- 1 cup quinoa, rinsed
- 2 cups water or vegetable broth
- 1 can (15 oz) black beans, drained and rinsed
- 1 cup corn kernels, fresh, canned, or frozen.
- 1/2 cup salsa
- 1 teaspoon ground cumin
- 1 teaspoon chili powder
- Salt, pepper, sliced green onions, lime wedges

Step by Step Preparations

Start by preheating your oven to 375°F (190°C). In a medium saucepan, bring water or vegetable broth to a boil. Add the quinoa, then decrease the heat to low, cover, and let it simmer for 15-20 minutes until the quinoa is cooked and the liquid is absorbed. Once done, remove from heat and allow it to cool somewhat.

In a large mixing bowl, combine the cooked quinoa with black beans, corn kernels, salsa, ground cumin, and chili powder. Season with salt and pepper to taste, ensuring everything is fully blended.

Arrange half bell peppers in a baking tray, placing them cut side up. Stuff each bell pepper half with the quinoa and black bean mixture, gently pushing down to compress it in.

Cover the baking dish with aluminum foil and bake in the preheated oven for 25-30 minutes until the bell peppers are cooked. Remove the foil and bake for a further 5 minutes, or until the tops are softly golden brown.

Once out of the oven, let the filled bell peppers cool for a few minutes before serving. Serve the filled bell peppers hot, garnishing with sliced green onions and lime wedges

---

Depending on availability and taste, use canned (drained and rinsed), frozen, or fresh corn. Salsa gives the stuffing mixture flavor and moisture; if you are sensitive to any particular ingredients, such as onion or garlic, use a low-FODMAP salsa.

Poultry, Meat and Potatoes

(Choose Low FODMAP Ingredients when necessary; The list in Appendices will guide you).

Grilled Chicken and Roasted Potatoes

Serving	Kcal	Carbs	Proteins	Fats	Fiber
4	350	30g	30g	12g	6g

Prep Time: 15 minutes
Cooking Time: 35 minutes
Total Time: 50 minutes

Ingredients

4 boneless, skinless chicken breasts

1 lb green beans, trimmed

1 lb baby potatoes, halved

2 tablespoons olive oil

2 cloves garlic, minced

1 teaspoon dried thyme

Salt and pepper

Step by Step Preparations

Start by preheating the grill to medium-high heat. In a large basin, mix the halved baby potatoes with 1 tablespoon of olive oil, chopped garlic, dried thyme, salt, and pepper. Toss the ingredients until the potatoes are equally covered.

Transfer the seasoned potatoes to a baking sheet lined with parchment paper, ensuring they are spread out in a single layer. Roast them in the preheated oven for 25-30 minutes, or until they attain a soft, golden brown texture, remembering to stir halfway through cooking.

While the potatoes are roasting, season the chicken breasts with salt and pepper. Grill them for 6-8 minutes each side, or until they are thoroughly cooked through and reach an internal temperature of 165°F (75°C). Once done, take them from the grill and allow them to rest for a few minutes before serving.

Meanwhile, in a different pot, bring water to a boil. Place the trimmed green beans in a steamer basket and cook them for 5-7 minutes, ensuring they stay soft but crisp.

Once all components are cooked to perfection, put the grilled chicken breasts, steaming green beans, and roasted potatoes on a serving plate.

Turkey Chili and Crushed Tomatoes

Serving	Kcal	Carbs	Proteins	Fats	Fiber
6	250	20g	20g	10g	6g

Prep Time: 15 minutes
Cooking Time: 30 minutes
Total Time: 45 minutes

Ingredients

- 1 lb ground turkey
- 1 onion, diced
- 2 bell peppers, diced
- 2 cloves garlic, minced
- 1 can (15 oz) kidney beans, drained and rinsed
- 1 can (15 oz) crushed tomatoes
- 1 cup vegetable broth
- 1 tablespoon olive oil
- 2 teaspoons chili powder
- 1 teaspoon ground cumin
- 1/2 teaspoon paprika
- Salt and pepper
- Fresh cilantro, sliced green onions
- Grated cheddar cheese, plain lactose-free yogurt or sour cream

Step by Step Preparations

In a large sized saucepan or Dutch oven, preheat the olive oil over medium heat. Introduce the chopped onion and bell peppers, letting them soften for around 5 minutes. Incorporate the minced garlic into the saucepan, letting it stew for a further minute until its scent fills the air.

Add the ground turkey to the saucepan, breaking it up with a spoon while it cooks. Continue heating until it browns and is well cooked through, 5-7 minutes. Sprinkle in the chili powder, powdered cumin, paprika, salt, and pepper, stirring to absorb the flavors for another minute until they become aromatic.

To the saucepan, add the drained and rinsed kidney beans, smashed tomatoes, and vegetable broth. Stir the ingredients until thoroughly blended.

Allow the chili to achieve a moderate simmer, then decrease the heat to low and let it simmer, uncovered, for 20-25 minutes. Stir periodically, ensuring the flavors merge together and the chili thickens to your desired consistency.

Taste the chili and adjust the spice as required. When ready to serve, garnish with fresh sliced green onions and shredded cheddar. For additional richness, try topping each dish with a dollop of plain lactose-free yogurt or sour cream.

Crushed tomatoes provide a full-bodied tomato taste without the indigestion-inducing acidity of raw tomatoes. Whether you want it with rice, cornbread, tortilla chips, or as a stand-alone dish, this turkey chili is sure to satisfy your need. Soluble fiber, which kidney beans contain, aids in bowel movement regulation and promotes digestive health.

Baked Turkey Meatballs and Spaghetti Squash

Serving	Kcal	Carbs	Proteins	Fats	Fiber
4	350	20g	25g	20g	6g

Prep Time: 20 minutes
Cooking Time: 40 minutes
Total Time: 1 hour

For the Turkey Meatballs

- 1 pound lean ground turkey
- 1/4 cup gluten-free breadcrumbs
- 1/4 cup grated Parmesan cheese
- 1 egg
- 2 cloves garlic, minced
- 2 tablespoons fresh parsley, chopped
- Salt and pepper

For the Marinara Sauce

- 1 can (14 oz) crushed tomatoes
- 1 tablespoon olive oil
- 2 cloves garlic, minced
- 1 teaspoon dried oregano
- 1 teaspoon dried basil
- Salt and pepper

For the Spaghetti Squash

- 1 medium spaghetti squash
- 1 tablespoon olive oil

- Salt and pepper

Step by Step Preparations

Start by preheating the oven to 400°F (200°C) and preparing a baking sheet either by coating it with parchment paper or by greasing it with olive oil.

Proceed by slicing the spaghetti squash in half lengthwise and scraping out the seeds. Brush the sliced sides with olive oil and season them with salt and pepper.

Arrange the squash halves cut-side down on the prepared baking sheet. Bake for 30-40 minutes, or until the squash is soft and readily punctured with a fork. Once cooked, apply a fork to scrape the meat into spaghetti-like strands. Set away for later use.

While the spaghetti squash is baking, use the chance to cook the turkey meatballs. In a spacious mixing basin, combine the ground turkey, gluten-free breadcrumbs, grated Parmesan cheese (if deciding to use), egg, minced garlic, chopped parsley, salt, and pepper. Ensure vigorous mixing until all elements are properly incorporated.

Shape the mixture into 1-inch meatballs and lay them on the prepared baking sheet. Bake in the preheated oven for 20-25 minutes, or until the meatballs are thoroughly cooked through and display a golden brown tone.

While the meatballs are baking, commence the preparation of the marinara sauce. In a saucepan, preheat the olive oil over medium heat. Add the minced garlic and sauté until fragrant, 1 minute.
Incorporate the smashed tomatoes, dried oregano, dry basil, salt, and pepper into the pot.

Allow the sauce to boil for 10-15 minutes, stirring regularly, until it gets a little thicker consistency. Once the meatballs have done baking, serve them steaming hot with the marinara sauce over the spaghetti squash noodles

Lemon Herb Roasted Chicken Thighs

Serving	Kcal	Carbs	Proteins	Fats	Fiber
4	450	35g	25g	20g	7g

Prep Time: 15 minutes
Cooking Time: 35 minutes
Total Time: 50 minutes

For Lemon Herb Roasted Chicken Thighs

- 4 bone-in, skin-on chicken thighs
- 2 tablespoons olive oil
- 2 cloves garlic, minced
- 1 tablespoon fresh lemon juice
- 1 teaspoon lemon zest
- 1 teaspoon dried thyme
- 1 teaspoon dried rosemary
- Salt and pepper

For Quinoa

- 1 cup quinoa, rinsed
- 2 cups water or chicken broth
- Salt

For Roasted Brussels Sprouts

- 1 pound Brussels sprouts, trimmed and halved
- 2 tablespoons olive oil
- Salt and pepper

Step by Step Preparations

Start by preheating the oven to 400°F (200°C). In a small bowl, combine together olive oil, minced garlic, lemon juice, lemon zest, dried thyme, dried rosemary, salt, and pepper to produce a delicious marinade for the chicken thighs.

Gently wipe the chicken thighs dry with paper towels, then put them in a baking dish. Generously brush both sides of the chicken thighs with the prepared marinade mixture.

Meanwhile, in a separate pot, bring water or low FODMAP chicken broth to a boil. Add the quinoa and salt, then decrease the heat to low. Cover and let it boil for approximately 15 minutes or until the quinoa is cooked and the liquid is absorbed.

Afterward, take it from the heat and let it rest for 5 minutes before fluffing it with a fork. On a baking sheet, sprinkle the Brussels sprouts with olive oil, salt, and pepper until equally covered. Spread them out in a single, equal layer on the baking sheet.

Once both the chicken thighs and Brussels sprouts are prepped, put them in the preheated oven. Roast for 25-30 minutes, or until the chicken is well cooked (with an internal temperature of 165°F or 75°C) and the Brussels sprouts are soft and caramelized to perfection.

Once cooked to perfection, gently remove the chicken thighs and Brussels sprouts from the oven. Serve the delicious lemon herb grilled chicken thighs atop the fluffy quinoa and delectably caramelized Brussels sprouts

For maximum flavor and moisture, go for bone-in, skin-on chicken thighs, which can be cooked ahead of time for meal prep or as a dinner option.

Chicken, Stir-Fry and Brown Rice

Serving	Kcal	Carbs	Proteins	Fats	Fiber
4	350	30g	25g	15g	5g

Prep Time: 15 minutes
Cooking Time: 15 minutes
Total Time: 30 minutes

Ingredients

- 1 lb boneless, skinless chicken breasts, thinly sliced
- 2 cups bell peppers, broccoli, snap peas, sliced
- 2 cloves garlic, minced
- 1 tablespoon fresh ginger, minced
- 2 tablespoons tamari sauce
- 2 tablespoons olive oil
- 2 cups cooked brown rice
- Salt and pepper
- Sesame seeds, sliced green onions

Step by Step Preparations

Start by heating 1 tablespoon of olive oil in a large pan or wok over medium-high heat. Add the cut chicken breasts and cook them until they lose their pink color in the middle, normally about 5-7 minutes. Once done, take the chicken from the pan and put it aside shortly.

In the same skillet, add the remaining tablespoon of olive oil. Incorporate the minced garlic and ginger, letting them to fry for 1 minute until they unleash their delicious scent.

Introduce the mixed veggies to the pan and stir-fry them for around 5 minutes, ensuring they attain a tender-crisp texture. Reintroduce the cooked chicken to the pan with the veggies.

Pour in the tamari sauce and stir everything up until completely incorporated. Allow the mixture to simmer for a further 1-2 minutes to ensure the chicken is cooked through. Season the stir-fry with salt and pepper to taste.

Serve the wonderful chicken and vegetable stir-fry over cooked brown rice. Garnish the dish with sesame seeds and chopped green onions

---

To keep the dish low in fat, use skinless, boneless chicken breasts; feel free to change the vegetables or source of protein as needed.

Turkey and Vegetable Soup

Serving	Kcal	Carbs	Proteins	Fats	Fiber
4	300	30g	20g	10g	4g

Prep Time: 15 minutes
Cooking Time: 30 minutes
Total Time: 45 minutes

Ingredients

- 1 tablespoon olive oil
- 1 pound ground turkey
- 1 onion, chopped
- 2 carrots, diced
- 2 stalks celery, diced
- 2 cloves garlic, minced
- 6 cups chicken or vegetable broth
- 2 cups rice noodles or quinoa noodles
- 2 cups spinach, chopped
- Salt and pepper

Step by Step Preparations

Begin by heating olive oil in a large saucepan over medium heat. Proceed to add the ground turkey and cook until it's beautifully browned, breaking it up with a spoon as it cooks.

Incorporate the chopped onion, carrots, celery, and minced garlic into the saucepan. Let them simmer for 5-7 minutes until they soften and become fragrant. Once the veggies have softened, add in the chicken or vegetable stock, and bring the soup to a vigorous boil.

Once the soup reaches a boiling temperature, put the gluten-free noodles into the saucepan. Lower the heat to medium-low and let the soup simmer for 10-12 minutes, or until the noodles are soft and cooked through.

After the noodles are done, add the chopped spinach to the saucepan and boil for an additional 2-3 minutes until the spinach wilts. Finally, season the soup with salt and pepper

Grilled Turkey Burger

Serving	Kcal	Carbs	Proteins	Fats	Fiber
4	300	20g	25g	14g	4g

Prep Time: 15 minutes
Cooking Time: 10 minutes
Total Time: 25 minutes

Ingredients

- 1 lb ground turkey
- 1/4 cup gluten-free breadcrumbs
- 1 egg
- 2 tablespoons fresh parsley, chopped
- 1 teaspoon garlic powder
- 1/2 teaspoon ground cumin
- Salt and pepper
- 4 gluten-free hamburger buns
- 4 leaves of lettuce
- 1 tomato, sliced
- 1 avocado, sliced

Step by Step Preparations

In a large mixing bowl, combine the ground turkey, gluten-free breadcrumbs, egg, chopped parsley, garlic powder, ground cumin, salt, and pepper. Mix until completely blended.

Divide the turkey mixture into 4 equal pieces and form each portion into a burger patty. Preheat your grill or grill pan to medium-high heat. Brush the grill grates with oil to avoid sticking.

Place the turkey burger patties on the grill and cook for 4-5 minutes each side, or until cooked through and no longer pink in the middle. While the burgers are cooking, gently toast the gluten-free hamburger buns on the grill.

To construct the burgers, lay a lettuce leaf on the bottom half of each bun, followed by a turkey burger patty, sliced tomato, and sliced avocado. Top with the other half of the bun.

For a gluten-free option, look for breadcrumbs made from rice or corn. For gluten-free buns, look for options made with tapioca starch, almond flour, or rice flour.

Chicken Caesar Salad and Dairy-Free Dressing

Serving	Kcal	Carbs	Proteins	Fats	Fiber
4	300	10g	25g	18g	4g

Prep Time: 15 minutes
Cooking Time: 20 minutes
Total Time: 35 minutes

For the Salad

- 2 boneless, skinless chicken breasts, cooked and sliced (or use pre-cooked chicken)
- 1 head romaine lettuce, washed and chopped
- 1 cup cherry tomatoes, halved
- 1/4 cup sliced black olives

For the Dairy-Free Caesar Dressing

- 1/2 cup dairy-free mayonnaise
- 2 tablespoons lemon juice
- 1 tablespoon Dijon mustard
- 2 cloves garlic, minced
- 1 teaspoon Worcestershire sauce
- Salt, pepper, water

Step by Step Preparations

Start by combining ground turkey, gluten-free breadcrumbs, egg, chopped parsley, garlic powder, ground cumin, salt, and pepper in a large mixing bowl. Mix well until all components are properly combined.

Divide the turkey mixture equally into 4 pieces, forming each portion into a burger patty. Preheat your grill or grill pan over medium-high heat, ensuring the grates are coated with oil to avoid sticking.

Once the grill is heated, lay the turkey burger patties on the grates and cook for 4-5 minutes each side, ensuring they are cooked through and no longer pink in the middle. While the burgers are cooking, gently toast the gluten-free hamburger buns on the grill until they attain a golden brown tint.

To build the burgers, start by laying a lettuce leaf on the bottom half of each bun, followed by a turkey burger patty, sliced tomato, and sliced avocado. Complete the construction by placing the second half of the bun on top.

Turkey and Avocado Wrap

Serving	Kcal	Carbs	Proteins	Fats	Fiber
2 wraps	350	35g	15g	18g	9g

Prep Time: 10 minutes
Cooking Time: 0 min.
Total Time: 10 minutes

Ingredients

- 2 large whole grain or gluten-free wraps
- 6 slices of low-sodium deli turkey breast
- 1 avocado, sliced
- 1 cup baby spinach leaves
- 1/2 cucumber, thinly sliced
- 1/4 cup hummus

Step by Step Preparations

Start by laying out the wraps evenly on a clean surface. Evenly distribute 2 tablespoons of hummus over each wrap, careful to leave a border around the edges.

Divide the young spinach leaves evenly between the two wraps, putting them at the middle of each wrap. Layer 3 slices of turkey breast onto the spinach on each wrap.

Distribute the sliced avocado and cucumber equally over the turkey pieces on each wrap. Fold in the sides of each wrap, then roll firmly from the bottom to produce a secure wrap. Before serving, cut each wrap in half diagonally for easy handling

Turkey breast from a low-sodium deli is a lean protein source that can aid in satiety and muscle repair without aggravating IBS symptoms.

Turkey and Vegetable Kabobs

Serving	Kcal	Carbs	Proteins	Fats	Fiber
4	250	20g	25g	9g	4g

Prep Time: 20 minutes
Cooking Time: 10 minutes
Total Time: 30 minutes

Ingredients

1 lb (450g) lean ground turkey

2 bell peppers, cut into chunks

2 zucchinis, sliced into rounds

1 cup pineapple chunks (fresh or canned in natural juice)

1 tablespoon olive oil

2 tablespoons barbecue sauce

Salt and pepper

Wooden or metal skewers

Step by Step Preparations

Start by preheating your grill to medium-high heat or by preheating your oven broiler. In a mixing bowl, combine the ground turkey, olive oil, low FODMAP barbecue sauce, salt, and pepper. Thoroughly mix until all components are well blended.

Divide the turkey mixture into 16 equal parts. Take one part and form it onto a skewer, alternating with chunks of bell pepper, slices of zucchini, and pineapple chunks. Repeat this method until all the turkey mixture and veggies are consumed, resulting in 4 skewers.

Place the skewers on the preheated grill or under the broiler. Cook for 4-5 minutes on each side, ensuring the turkey is well cooked through and the veggies are soft with a small sear.

Once cooked, take the skewers from the grill or broiler and let them rest for a few minutes before serving.

For a full dinner, these kabobs can be served as the main course with cooked quinoa or a side salad.

Grilled Steak and Mashed Sweet Potatoes

Serving	Kcal	Carbs	Proteins	Fats	Fiber
4	450	20g	30g	25g	5g

Prep Time: 15 minutes
Cooking Time: 40 minutes
Total Time: 55 minutes

For the Grilled Steak

- 4 sirloin steaks (about 6 oz each), trimmed of excess fat
- 2 tablespoons olive oil
- 2 cloves garlic, minced
- Salt and pepper to taste

For the Roasted Asparagus

- 1 bunch asparagus, tough ends trimmed
- 2 tablespoons olive oil
- Salt and pepper

For the Mashed Sweet Potatoes

- 2 large sweet potatoes, peeled and cubed
- 2 tablespoons unsalted butter or olive oil
- 1/4 cup lactose-free milk or vegetable broth
- Salt and pepper

Step by Step Preparations

Start by blending olive oil, minced garlic, salt, and pepper in a small bowl. Thoroughly massage the mixture over the steaks, ensuring uniform covering. Allow them to marinade for a minimum of 15 minutes while you prepare the other dinner components.

Preheat the grill to medium-high heat. Grill the steaks for 4-5 minutes each side, or until they achieve your chosen amount of doneness. Once done, remove them from the fire and let them rest for a few minutes before serving.

Simultaneously, preheat the oven to 400°F (200°C). Arrange the trimmed asparagus stalks on a baking sheet. Drizzle with olive oil and season with salt and pepper, tossing them to coat evenly. Roast the asparagus in the preheated oven for 12-15 minutes, or until they become tender with a little crispiness.

Meanwhile, lay the diced sweet potatoes in a big saucepan and fill them with water. Bring the saucepan to a boil over medium-high heat, then decrease the heat to medium-low and let it simmer for 15-20 minutes, or until the sweet potatoes are easily pierced with a fork.

Once the sweet potatoes are done, drain them and return them to the saucepan. Add butter or olive oil, lactose-free milk or vegetable broth, salt, and pepper.

Using a potato masher, mash the sweet potatoes until they attain a smooth and creamy consistency. Adjust the seasoning

---

Lean meats such as sirloin steak are high in iron and protein, and eating them can help lower fat intake and lessen symptoms of IBS.

Beef with Broccoli

Serving	Kcal	Carbs	Proteins	Fats	Fiber
4	300	15g	25g	15g	5g

Prep Time: 20 minutes
Cooking Time: 15 minutes
Total Time: 35 minutes

Ingredients

- 1 lb (450g) lean beef steak, thinly sliced against the grain
- 2 cups broccoli florets
- 1 red bell pepper, sliced
- 1 yellow bell pepper, sliced
- 1 cup snow peas, trimmed
- 2 cloves garlic, minced
- 2 tablespoons low-sodium soy sauce or tamari
- 1 tablespoon rice vinegar
- 1 tablespoon sesame oil
- 1 tablespoon cornstarch
- 1 tablespoon olive oil
- Salt and pepper
- Cooked rice or quinoa
- Sesame seeds, sliced green onions

Step by Step Preparations

In a small bowl, mix the low-sodium soy sauce or tamari, rice vinegar, sesame oil, and cornstarch to make the stir-fry sauce. Set away for later use.

Warm the olive oil in a large pan or wok over medium-high heat. Add the minced garlic and sauté for 1 minute until it gets aromatic.

Introduce the thinly sliced beef to the pan and stir-fry for 2-3 minutes until it browns and cooks through fully. Once done, take the steak from the pan and put it aside.

In the same pan, add the broccoli florets, sliced bell peppers, and snow peas. Stir-fry the veggies for 3-4 minutes until they acquire a tender-crisp texture.

Reintroduce the cooked meat to the pan with the veggies. Pour the prepared stir-fry sauce over the meat and veggies, ensuring complete covering by tossing well.

Allow the mixture to simmer for a further 1-2 minutes until the sauce slightly thickens and everything is cooked through.
Season the meal with salt and pepper according to taste preferences.

Serve the fragrant stir-fry hot, possibly over cooked rice or quinoa. Garnish with sesame seeds and sliced green onions

---

When you're looking for a quick and easy dinner option that's satisfying and nutritious, this stir-fry is perfect for busy weeknights because it can be customized with your favorite vegetables or protein sources.

Beef and Bean Chili

Serving	Kcal	Carbs	Proteins	Fats	Fiber
4	350	30g	25g	15g	8g

Prep Time: 15 minutes
Cooking Time: 30 minutes
Total Time: 45 minutes

Ingredients

- 1 pound lean ground beef
- 1 can (15 oz) black beans, drained and rinsed
- 1 can (14.5 oz) diced tomatoes
- 1 cup corn kernels (fresh, frozen, or canned)
- 1 onion, diced
- 2 cloves garlic, minced
- 1 bell pepper, diced
- 1 tablespoon chili powder
- 1 teaspoon ground cumin
- 1/2 teaspoon paprika
- 1/4 teaspoon cayenne pepper
- Salt and pepper
- 1 tablespoon olive oil

Step by Step Preparations

Begin by heating olive oil in a big saucepan or Dutch oven over medium heat. Introduce the chopped onion and bell pepper, cooking until they soften, 5 minutes.

Incorporate the minced garlic into the saucepan and heat for a further 1-2 minutes till it emits its pungent scent. Proceed to add the ground beef to the saucepan, using a spoon to break it apart as it cooks, getting a lovely browned texture in approximately 5-7 minutes.

Stir in the chili powder, ground cumin, paprika, and cayenne pepper if desired. Cook the mixture for 1 minute, stirring regularly, until the spices become aromatic.

Add the chopped tomatoes along with their juices, black beans, and corn to the saucepan. Stir everything together to ensure complete combination.

Bring the chili to a light simmer, then decrease the heat to a simmering point and let it stew uncovered for approximately 20-25 minutes. Remember to stir periodically to enable the flavors to mingle and the chili to thicken to your preferred consistency. Finally, season the chili with salt and pepper

---

If you are allergic to onion or garlic, choose canned tomatoes that don't have any added ingredient.

Lamb Kebabs and Quinoa Tabbouleh

Serving	Kcal	Carbs	Proteins	Fats	Fiber
4	450	30g	25g	25g	7g

Prep Time: 20 minutes
Marinating Time: 30 minute
Cooking Time: 10 minutes
Total Time: 1 hour

For Lamb Kebabs

- 1 lb lamb, cubed
- 1 tablespoon olive oil
- 2 cloves garlic, minced
- 1 teaspoon dried oregano
- Salt and pepper
- Metal or wooden skewers

For Greek Salad

- 2 tomatoes, diced
- 1 cucumber, diced
- 1/2 red onion, thinly sliced
- 1/4 cup Kalamata olives, pitted and halved
- 1/4 cup crumbled feta cheese
- 2 tablespoons extra virgin olive oil
- 1 tablespoon red wine vinegar
- 1 teaspoon dried oregano
- Salt and pepper

For Quinoa Tabbouleh

- 1 cup cooked quinoa, cooled
- 1 cup parsley, chopped
- 1/4 cup mint leaves, chopped
- 1 tomato, diced
- 1/4 cup cucumber, diced
- 1/4 cup green onions, thinly sliced
- 2 tablespoons lemon juice
- 2 tablespoons extra virgin olive oil
- Salt and pepper

Step by Step Preparations

For Lamb Kebabs

Start by combining together olive oil, minced garlic, dried oregano, salt, and pepper in a basin. Add the cubed lamb to the marinade, ensuring each piece is equally covered.

Allow the lamb to marinade in the refrigerator for a minimum of 30 minutes, or prolong the marinating period to up to 4 hours if your schedule permits. Thread the marinated lamb onto skewers.

Preheat a grill or grill pan over medium-high heat. Grill the lamb kebabs for 3-4 minutes on each side, or until they achieve your chosen amount of doneness.

For Greek Salad

In a spacious bowl, mix together the diced tomatoes, cucumber, red onion, Kalamata olives, and crumbled feta cheese. In a separate small bowl, mix together the extra virgin olive oil, red wine vinegar, dried oregano, salt, and pepper to make the dressing. Drizzle the dressing over the salad mixture and gently toss to achieve uniform covering. Set the salad aside.

For the Quinoa Tabbouleh

Combine the cooked quinoa, chopped parsley, chopped mint leaves, diced tomato, diced cucumber, and sliced green onions in a large bowl.

In another small dish, mix together the lemon juice, extra virgin olive oil, salt, and pepper to create the dressing. Pour the dressing over the quinoa tabbouleh and carefully toss to include all ingredients.

To serve, dish out the lamb kebabs, Greek salad, and quinoa tabbouleh onto individual serving plates.

Beef and Mushroom Stroganoff

Serving	Kcal	Carbs	Proteins	Fats	Fiber
4	450	40g	30g	18g	3g

Prep Time: 15 minutes
Cooking Time: 25 minutes
Total Time: 40 minutes

Ingredients

- 8 oz rice or quinoa pasta
- 1 lb lean beef, thinly sliced, sirloin or tenderloin
- 8 oz mushrooms, sliced
- 1 onion, finely chopped
- 2 cloves garlic, minced
- 1 cup beef broth
- 1 cup lactose-free sour cream or coconut cream
- 2 tablespoons gluten-free all-purpose flour
- 2 tablespoons olive oil
- 1 tablespoon Worcestershire sauce
- Salt and pepper

Step by Step Preparations

Begin by cooking the gluten-free pasta following the directions on the box. Once cooked, rinse the pasta and keep it away for later use.

In a large skillet, heat the olive oil over medium-high heat. Add the thinly sliced beef and heat until it acquires a golden brown color on both sides, 3-4 minutes. Remove the steak from the pan and put it aside shortly.

In the same skillet, mix the sliced mushrooms and chopped onion. Cook until the mushrooms become soft and the onions become translucent, which normally takes around 5-6 minutes.

Introduce the minced garlic to the pan, frying for a further 1-2 minutes until it emits its delicious scent. Sprinkle the gluten-free all-purpose flour over the mushroom and onion mixture, ensuring thorough mixing. Cook for another 1-2 minutes to eradicate any raw flour flavor.

Gradually add in the low FODMAP beef broth while stirring continually to avoid lumps from developing. Allow the mixture to come to a medium simmer.

Return the cooked beef to the pan, followed by tossing in the lactose-free sour cream (or coconut cream) and Worcestershire sauce. Let the mixture boil for another 5 minutes, stirring regularly, until the sauce gets a little thicker consistency.

Adjust the seasoning with salt and pepper according to taste preferences. Serve over the cooked gluten-free spaghetti

---

The whole family will find this beef and mushroom stroganoff to be a delicious supper option.

Beef and Cabbage Soup

Serving	Kcal	Carbs	Proteins	Fats	Fiber
4	300	25g	25g	10g	5g

Prep Time: 15 minutes
Cooking Time: 45 minutes
Total Time: 1 hour

Ingredients

- 1 pound lean beef stew meat, cut into bite-sized pieces
- 4 cups beef broth
- 2 cups cabbage, shredded
- 2 carrots, diced
- 2 stalks celery, diced
- 2 potatoes, peeled and diced
- 1 onion, chopped
- 2 cloves garlic, minced
- 1 tablespoon olive oil
- 1 teaspoon dried thyme
- Salt and pepper

Step by Step Preparations

Begin by heating olive oil in a large saucepan over medium heat. Introduce the chopped onion and minced garlic, cooking until they soften, 3-4 minutes.

Add the beef stew meat to the saucepan, ensuring to brown it on both sides, which should take around 5-7 minutes. Incorporate the diced carrots, celery, and potatoes into the saucepan, simmering for a further 5 minutes.

Proceed to pour in the beef broth and add the dried thyme, bringing the soup to a boil.

Next, add the shredded cabbage to the saucepan, stirring to mix all ingredients completely. Allow the soup to boil for 30-35 minutes, ensuring the veggies become soft and the meat cooks through. Finally, season the soup with salt and pepper

Pork Tenderloin with Roasted Root Vegetables

Serving	Kcal	Carbs	Proteins	Fats	Fiber
4	400	35g	30g	15g	5g

Prep Time: 15 minutes
Cooking Time: 40 minutes
Total Time: 55 minutes

Ingredients

- 1 lb pork tenderloin
- 2 cups carrots, parsnips, and potatoes, diced
- 1 tablespoon olive oil
- 1 teaspoon dried thyme
- 1 teaspoon dried rosemary
- Salt and pepper
- 1 cup wild rice, rinsed
- 2 cups chicken or vegetable broth

Step by Step Preparations

Preheat your oven to 400°F (200°C) to ensure it's ready for the following stage. In a big dish, sprinkle the diced root veggies with olive oil, dried thyme, dry rosemary, salt, and pepper until each piece is fully coated.

Spread the seasoned root veggies equally on a baking sheet lined with parchment paper. Place the sheet in the preheated oven and let the veggies roast for 25-30 minutes until they're soft and acquire a mild caramelization.

While the veggies are roasting, prepare the wild rice. Bring the low FODMAP chicken or vegetable broth to a boil in a medium saucepan. Add the washed wild rice, then decrease the heat to low, cover, and let it simmer for 30-35 minutes until the rice is cooked and the liquid is absorbed. After simmering, remove the pot from heat and let it remain covered for 5 minutes before fluffing the rice with a fork.

Season the pork tenderloin with salt and pepper on both sides.
In a skillet over medium-high heat, add a sprinkle of olive oil. Once the pan is heated, sear the pork tenderloin on both sides until it acquires a golden brown hue, 2-3 minutes per side.

Transfer the seared pork tenderloin to a baking dish and roast it in the preheated oven for 15-20 minutes, or until the internal temperature reaches 145°F (63°C) for medium doneness. Once done, take the pork tenderloin from the oven and allow it to rest for 5 minutes before slicing. Serve the delicious pork tenderloin with the roasted root vegetables and wild rice.

Meatloaf and Steamed Green Beans

Serving	Kcal	Carbs	Proteins	Fats	Fiber
4	350	15g	25g	20g	5g

Prep Time: 20 minutes
Cooking Time: 1 hour
Total Time: 1 hour and 20 minutes

For the Meatloaf

- 1 pound lean ground turkey or beef
- 1/2 cup gluten-free breadcrumbs
- 1 egg
- 1/4 cup ketchup
- 1 tablespoon Worcestershire sauce
- 1 teaspoon dried oregano
- 1 teaspoon dried thyme
- Salt and pepper

For the Cauliflower Mash

- 1 medium head cauliflower, chopped into florets
- 2 tablespoons lactose-free milk or unsweetened almond milk
- 2 tablespoons olive oil
- Salt and pepper

For the Steamed Green Beans

- 2 cups green beans, trimmed

- Water, salt

Step by Step Preparations

Start by preheating your oven to 375°F (190°C) and gently coating a loaf pan with cooking spray or oil.

In a spacious mixing basin, combine the ground turkey or beef, gluten-free breadcrumbs, egg, low FODMAP ketchup, Worcestershire sauce, dried oregano, dried thyme, salt, and pepper. Mix the ingredients well until properly blended.

Transfer the beef mixture into the prepared loaf pan and form it into a loaf. Bake the meatloaf in the preheated oven for 45-50 minutes, or until it's cooked through and the internal temperature reaches 160°F (71°C).

While the meatloaf is baking, start to create the cauliflower mash. Steam the cauliflower florets until they are soft, 10-12 minutes. Drain out any surplus water.

Transfer the cooked cauliflower to a food processor and add the lactose-free milk, olive oil, salt, and pepper. Blend the ingredients until they become smooth and creamy. Adjust the seasoning to your taste preferences.

Simultaneously, steam the green beans until they achieve a tender consistency, which normally takes around 5-7 minutes. Season them with salt according to your taste.

Once the meatloaf is entirely cooked, remove it from the oven and allow it to rest for a few minutes before slicing. To serve, place the sliced meatloaf beside a hearty serving of cauliflower mash and cooked green beans on the side.

Beef and Basmati Rice

Serving	Kcal	Carbs	Proteins	Fats	Fiber
4	400	10g	25g	30g	3g

Prep Time: 20 minutes
Cooking Time: 40 minutes
Total Time: 1 hour

Ingredients

- 1 lb beef sirloin or stew meat, cut into bite-sized pieces
- 1 can (14 oz) coconut milk
- 2 cups bell peppers, carrots, and green beans, diced
- 1 onion, finely chopped
- 2 cloves garlic, minced
- 1 tablespoon ginger, minced
- 2 tablespoons curry powder
- 1 teaspoon ground cumin
- 1 teaspoon ground coriander
- 1/2 teaspoon turmeric powder
- 1 tablespoon olive oil
- Salt and pepper
- Cooked basmati rice

Step by Step Preparations

In a big skillet or saucepan, warm up the olive oil over a medium temperature. Toss in the chopped onion and let it sear until it becomes translucent, which should take roughly 3-4 minutes.

Introduce the minced garlic and ginger to the pan, and let them combine for another 1-2 minutes until their tempting scent fills the air.

Now, add the beef to the pan and let it sizzle until it's browned on both sides, which should take around 5-7 minutes of sautéing.

Sprinkle in the curry powder, powdered cumin, ground coriander, and turmeric powder. Leave them in the pan for about a minute, swirling regularly until they're toasted and unleash their delicious smell.

Next, pour in the coconut milk and give everything a good swirl to combine the flavors. Allow the mixture to gradually simmer. Add the medley of mixed veggies to the pan and let them simmer for approximately 15-20 minutes, or until the beef achieves a soft condition and the vegetables are well cooked.

To optimize the flavor, season with salt and pepper according to your taste. When everything is done, serve over a bed of prepared basmati rice.

Pork Stir-Fry with Bell Peppers

Serving	Kcal	Carbs	Proteins	Fats	Fiber
4	300	15g	25g	15g	4g

Prep Time: 15 minutes
Cooking Time: 15 minutes
Total Time: 30 minutes

Ingredients

- 1 lb pork tenderloin, thinly sliced
- 2 bell peppers, sliced
- 1 cup snow peas, trimmed
- 1 can (8 oz) sliced water chestnuts, drained
- 3 cloves garlic, minced
- 2 tablespoons low-sodium soy sauce or tamari
- 1 tablespoon rice vinegar
- 1 tablespoon sesame oil
- 1 tablespoon cornstarch
- 2 tablespoons olive oil or vegetable oil
- Salt and pepper
- Cooked rice or quinoa

Step by Step Preparations

Start by mixing together soy sauce, rice vinegar, sesame oil, and cornstarch in a small bowl to produce the sauce. Set it away for later use.

In a generous-sized pan or wok, heat 1 tablespoon of olive oil over medium-high heat. Introduce the sliced pork, stir-frying until it browns and cooks through, 3-4 minutes. Once done, take the pork from the pan and put it aside shortly.

In the same skillet, add the remaining tablespoon of olive oil. Incorporate the minced garlic, stir-frying for around 30 seconds until it exudes an aromatic scent.

Next, add the sliced bell peppers, snow peas, and water chestnuts to the pan. Stir-fry the veggies for around 3-4 minutes until they achieve a crisp-tender stage.

Reintroduce the cooked pork to the pan with the veggies. Pour the prepared sauce over the meat and veggies, ensuring uniform covering by tossing everything together. Allow it to simmer for another 1-2 minutes until the sauce thickens slightly.

Season the meal with salt and pepper according to taste preferences. Serve over cooked rice or quinoa

Baked Potato and Steamed Broccoli

Serving	Kcal	Carbs	Proteins	Fats	Fiber
4	250	45g	5g	6g	6g

Prep Time: 10 minutes
Cooking Time: 45 minutes
Total Time: 55 minutes

Ingredients

- 4 medium-sized russet potatoes
- 1 cup coconut milk or almond-based sour cream
- 1/4 cup fresh chives, chopped
- 2 cups broccoli florets
- 1 tablespoon olive oil
- Salt and pepper

Step by Step Preparations

Begin by preheating your oven to 400°F (200°C). Thoroughly clean the potatoes under running water and dry them with a kitchen towel.
Using a fork, puncture each potato several times to encourage steam escape while baking.

Place the potatoes directly on the oven rack or on a baking sheet coated with parchment paper. Bake them for 45-60 minutes until they are soft when pricked with a fork.

While the potatoes are roasting, steam the broccoli florets until cooked, which normally takes approximately 5-7 minutes. You may use either a steamer basket or a microwave-safe dish with a little water covered with plastic wrap for steaming.

Once the potatoes are roasted, take them from the oven and allow them to cool gently for a few minutes. To serve, slice each potato open lengthwise and fluff the insides with a fork.

Top each potato with a dollop of dairy-free sour cream, steaming broccoli florets, and chopped chives. Drizzle olive oil over the top and season with salt and pepper to taste. Serve immediately when still hot.

Mashed Potatoes

Serving	Kcal	Carbs	Proteins	Fats	Fiber
4	200	30g	3g	8g	3g

Prep Time: 10 minutes
Cooking Time: 20 minutes
Total Time: 30 minutes

Ingredients

- 4 large potatoes (about 2 pounds), peeled and cut into chunks
- 1/4 cup coconut oil or olive oil spread
- 1/2 cup unsweetened almond milk
- Salt and pepper

Step by Step Preparations

Commence by putting the potato pieces in a big saucepan and filling them with cold water, adding a pinch of salt to the water.

Bring the water to a vigorous boil over high heat, then decrease the heat to medium-low and allow the potatoes to simmer for 15-20 minutes until they attain a fork-tender texture.

Once cooked, drain the potatoes completely and return them to the saucepan. Incorporate the dairy-free butter and almond milk into the saucepan with the cooked potatoes.

Utilize a potato masher or fork to mash the potatoes till they become smooth and creamy, altering the consistency with extra almond milk if required. Season the mashed potatoes with salt and pepper

Roasted Potato Wedges and Herbs

Serving	Kcal	Carbs	Proteins	Fats	Fiber
4	200	30g	4g	8g	4g

Prep Time: 10 minutes
Cooking Time: 30 minutes
Total Time: 40 minutes

Ingredients

- 4 medium potatoes, scrubbed and cut into wedges
- 2 tablespoons olive oil
- 2 cloves garlic, minced
- 1 teaspoon dried thyme
- 1 teaspoon dried rosemary
- Salt and pepper

Step by Step Preparations

Preheat your oven to 425°F (220°C) and prepare a baking sheet by lining it with parchment paper. In a wide mixing basin, combine the potato wedges with olive oil, chopped garlic, dried thyme, dried rosemary, salt, and pepper, ensuring a uniform coating.

Arrange the seasoned potato wedges in a single layer on the prepared baking sheet. Roast the potato wedges in the preheated oven for 25-30 minutes, remembering to rotate them halfway during the cooking time.

They should reach a golden brown, crispy surface and a soft inside when done. Once done, take the potato wedges from the oven and transfer them to a serving platter.

Potato Salad with Dijon Mustard Dressing

Serving	Kcal	Carbs	Proteins	Fats	Fiber
4	250	30g	3g	13g	4g

Prep Time: 15 minutes
Cooking Time: 20 minutes
Total Time: 35 minutes

Ingredients

- 1 1/2 lbs potatoes, Yukon Gold or red potatoes, washed and diced
- 2 stalks celery, diced
- 1/2 red onion, finely chopped
- 1/4 cup fresh parsley, chopped

Dijon Mustard Dressing

- 1/4 cup olive oil
- 2 tablespoons Dijon mustard
- 2 tablespoons apple cider vinegar
- 1 tablespoon maple syrup
- Salt and pepper

Step by Step Preparations

Begin by putting the diced potatoes in a substantially sized saucepan and filling them with water. Bring the saucepan to a vigorous boil over high heat, then decrease the heat to medium-low and allow the potatoes to simmer for 15-20 minutes, or until they reach a fork-tender consistency.

While the potatoes are cooking, use the time to create the Dijon mustard dressing. In a small bowl, mix together the olive oil, Dijon mustard, apple cider vinegar, and, if preferred, maple syrup. Season the mixture with salt and pepper, ensuring complete integration until a cohesive dressing is created.

Once the potatoes have finished cooking, rinse them and allow them to cool somewhat. In a large mixing basin, combine the cooked potatoes with the diced celery, chopped red onion, and fresh parsley.

Drizzle the prepared Dijon mustard dressing over the potato mixture, gently tossing until each component is uniformly covered. To guarantee ideal flavor, taste the salad and adjust the spice

Sweet Potato Hash with and Spinach

Serving	Kcal	Carbs	Proteins	Fats	Fiber
4	200	30g	3g	9g	5g

Prep Time: 15 minutes
Cooking Time: 25 minutes
Total Time: 40 minutes

Ingredients

- 2 large sweet potatoes, peeled and diced into small cubes
- 1 bell pepper, diced
- 1 onion, diced
- 2 cups spinach leaves, chopped
- 2 tablespoons olive oil
- 1 teaspoon paprika
- 1/2 teaspoon garlic powder
- Salt and pepper

Step by Step Preparations

Begin by heating the olive oil in a suitably sized pan over medium heat.

Introduce the diced sweet potatoes to the pan and let them simmer for 10-12 minutes, turning periodically, until they achieve a soft, lightly browned condition.

Incorporate the chopped bell pepper and onion into the pan with the sweet potatoes. Continue cooking for another 5-7 minutes, until the veggies attain a softened texture.

Add the chopped spinach to the pan, tossing it in well. Cook for a further 2-3 minutes until the spinach wilts. Sprinkle the paprika and garlic powder evenly over the hash, then season with salt and pepper according to your taste preferences. Stir the mixture carefully to ensure the flavors merge together.

Continue cooking the hash for a further 3-5 minutes, or until all the veggies are well cooked through.

Potato and Leek Soup

Serving	Kcal	Carbs	Proteins	Fats	Fiber
4	300	30g	4g	20g	3g

Prep Time: 15 minutes
Cooking Time: 30 minutes
Total Time: 45 minutes

Ingredients

- 2 tablespoons olive oil
- 2 leeks, white and light green parts only, sliced
- 3 medium potatoes, peeled and diced
- 4 cups vegetable broth
- 1 can (14 oz) coconut milk
- Salt and pepper

Step by Step Preparations

In a spacious saucepan, warm the olive oil over medium heat. Add the sliced leeks and sauté for 5 minutes until they become soft. Incorporate the diced potatoes into the saucepan and continue cooking for another 3-4 minutes, stirring regularly to achieve equal cooking.

Pour in the veggie broth and bring the mixture to a mild boil. Reduce the heat to low, cover the saucepan, and allow it to simmer for around 15-20 minutes until the potatoes are soft and tender.

Once the potatoes have achieved the correct consistency, take the saucepan from the heat and allow it to cool slightly. Using either an immersion blender or a normal blender, slowly mix the soup until it gets a smooth, creamy texture.

If using a conventional blender, return the pureed soup to the saucepan and set it back over low heat. Stir in the coconut milk and let the soup cook through. Finally, season the soup with salt and pepper

Scalloped Potatoes and Yeast

Serving	Kcal	Carbs	Proteins	Fats	Fiber
6	200	30g	5g	7g	4g

Prep Time: 15 minutes
Cooking Time: 1 hour
Total Time: 1 hour 15 minutes

Ingredients

- 2 lbs Yukon Gold potatoes, thinly sliced
- 1 onion, thinly sliced
- 2 cloves garlic, minced
- 2 cups unsweetened almond milk
- 1/4 cup nutritional yeast
- 2 tablespoons olive oil
- 2 tablespoons all-purpose flour
- 1 teaspoon Dijon mustard
- 1/2 teaspoon dried thyme
- Salt and pepper

Step by Step Preparations

Start by preheating your oven to 375°F (190°C) and gently greasing a 9x13-inch baking dish with olive oil or cooking spray.

In a small saucepan over medium heat, warm the olive oil. Add the minced garlic and sliced onion, cooking until the onion turns soft and translucent, often approximately 5 minutes.

Then, whisk in the flour and continue cooking for an additional 1-2 minutes, stirring frequently to produce a roux. Gradually mix in the almond milk, nutritional yeast, Dijon mustard, dried thyme, salt, and pepper. Keep stirring frequently until the sauce thickens, which normally takes around 5-7 minutes.

Now, place a layer of thinly sliced potatoes in the bottom of the prepared baking dish. Pour some of the dairy-free cheese sauce over the potatoes, spreading them evenly with a spatula.

Repeat the stacking technique with the remaining potatoes and sauce until all are utilized, culminating with a layer of sauce on top.
Cover the baking dish with aluminum foil and bake in the preheated oven for 45 minutes.

After 45 minutes, remove the cover and continue baking for an additional 15-20 minutes, or until the potatoes become soft and the top turns golden brown and bubbling. Once done, take the scalloped potatoes out of the oven and allow them to cool for a few minutes before serving.

Hasselback Potatoes with Rosemary

Serving	Kcal	Carbs	Proteins	Fats	Fiber
4	180	26g	3g	8g	3g

Prep Time: 15 minutes
Cooking Time: 45 minutes
Total Time: 1 hour

Ingredients

- 4 medium-sized potatoes, Yukon Gold or Russet
- 2 tablespoons olive oil
- 2 tablespoons fresh rosemary, finely chopped
- Salt and pepper

Step by Step Preparations

Begin by properly washing and cleaning the potatoes under cold water. Once washed, blot them dry with a clean kitchen towel.

Place one potato on a chopping board. Starting from one end, lightly make small slices across the potato, ensuring not to cut all the way through. Leave 1/8 inch (3 mm) intact at the bottom of the potato. Repeat this step with the remaining potatoes.

Arrange the sliced potatoes on a baking sheet coated with parchment paper or aluminum foil.

Drizzle the olive oil over the potatoes, ensuring it seeps between the pieces. Utilize a pastry brush or your hands to evenly coat each potato with olive oil.

Sprinkle the chopped rosemary over the potatoes, carefully pushing it into the slices to achieve uniform distribution.
Generously season the potatoes with salt and pepper.

Bake in the preheated oven for 40-45 minutes, or until the potatoes display a golden brown color and attain a crispy texture on the outside, while remaining fork-tender in the core. Serve as a side dish or appetizer.

Potato Pancakes

Serving	Kcal	Carbs	Proteins	Fats	Fiber
4	200	25g	4g	8g	2g

Prep Time: 15 minutes
Cooking Time: 20 minutes
Total Time: 35 minutes

Ingredients

- 2 large potatoes, peeled and grated
- 1/2 cup gluten-free all-purpose flour
- 2 tablespoons chives, finely chopped
- 1 egg, lightly beaten
- 1/4 teaspoon salt
- 1/4 teaspoon black pepper
- 2-3 tablespoons olive oil
- Sour cream or Greek yogurt

Step by Step Preparations

Begin by putting the shredded potatoes in a clean kitchen towel and carefully squeezing out any excess moisture. In a spacious mixing basin, add the grated potatoes, gluten-free flour, chopped chives, beaten egg, salt, and black pepper, stirring until fully incorporated.

Warm 1 tablespoon of olive oil in a large non-stick pan over medium heat. Take 1/4 cup of the potato mixture and form it into a pancake. Carefully set it in the skillet and flatten gently with a spatula.

Repeat this method with the remaining potato mixture, frying 3-4 pancakes at a time depending on the size of your skillet. Ensure not to overcrowd the pan.

Cook the pancakes for 3-4 minutes on each side, or until they attain a beautiful golden brown color and crispy texture. Once done, remove the pancakes from the skillet to a dish lined with paper towels to absorb any leftover oil.

Continue this procedure with the remaining potato mixture, adding extra olive oil to the pan as required. Serve the scrumptious potato pancakes with a dab of sour cream or Greek yogurt on top

Potato and Vegetable Frittata

Serving	Kcal	Carbs	Proteins	Fats	Fiber
4	250	20g	12g	14g	3g

Prep Time: 15 minutes
Cooking Time: 25 minutes
Total Time: 40 minutes

Ingredients

- 6 large eggs
- 2 medium potatoes, peeled and diced
- 1 bell pepper, diced
- 1 small onion, diced
- 1 cup spinach leaves, chopped
- 1/2 cup vegan cheddar or mozzarella, shredded
- 2 tablespoons olive oil
- Salt and pepper

Step by Step Preparations

Preheat your oven to 375°F (190°C) to get it ready for the following stages. In a wide oven-safe pan, heat up the olive oil over medium heat. Introduce the diced potatoes and simmer them for 5 minutes, stirring periodically, until they start to soften.

Incorporate the chopped bell pepper and onion (if using) into the pan and continue cooking for another 3-4 minutes until the veggies achieve a soft stage.

Meanwhile, in a separate dish, rapidly whisk together the eggs until they are completely beaten. Season the mixture with salt and pepper according to your taste.

Carefully pour the whisked eggs over the cooked veggies in the pan, maintaining a uniform distribution. Next, sprinkle the chopped spinach equally over the top of the egg mixture, followed by the dairy-free cheese.

Allow the frittata to cook on the stovetop for 3-4 minutes, monitoring as the edges begin to firm. Once the sides have formed, move the pan to the preheated oven and bake for 15-20 minutes, or until the frittata is completely set in the middle and develops a gently golden brown tint on top.

Upon completion of baking, remove the pan from the oven and allow the frittata to cool for a few minutes before slicing and serving.

IBS friendly Breakfast and Brunch Recipes

Scrambled eggs with spinach

Serving	Kcal	Carbs	Proteins	Fats	Fiber
2	180	5g	12g	13g	2g

Prep Time: 5 minutes
Cooking Time: 10 minutes
Total Time: 15 minutes

Ingredients

- 4 large eggs
- 1 cup fresh spinach leaves, chopped
- 1 medium tomato, diced
- 1 tablespoon olive oil or butter
- Salt and pepper

Step by Step Preparations

In a bowl, whisk the eggs well until they are well beaten, then season with salt and pepper according to your taste. In a non-stick skillet over medium heat, heat up the olive oil or butter until it's ready.

Introduce the diced tomato to the pan and let it simmer for 2-3 minutes until it slightly softens. Add the chopped spinach to the pan and continue cooking for another 1-2 minutes until it wilts. Pour the beaten eggs into the pan over the spinach and tomatoes.

Allow the eggs to boil undisturbed for a minute or two until they start setting around the edges. Using a spatula, gently whisk the eggs, moving them from the borders towards the center of the pan, until they achieve your chosen consistency.

Once the eggs are thoroughly cooked, remove the pan from the heat and place the scrambled eggs onto plates for dishing.

Grilled chicken salad and olive oil vinaigrette

Serving	Kcal	Carbs	Proteins	Fats	Fiber
4	250	10g	25g	12g	3g

Prep Time: 15 minutes
Cooking Time: 15 minutes
Total Time: 30 minutes

Ingredients

- 2 boneless, skinless chicken breasts
- 6 cups spinach, arugula, and romaine
- 1 cucumber, sliced
- 1/4 cup cherry tomatoes, halved
- 1/4 cup sliced red onion
- 1/4 cup sliced black olives
- 2 tablespoons olive oil
- 1 tablespoon red wine vinegar
- 1 teaspoon Dijon mustard
- Salt and pepper

Step by Step Preparations

Start by preheating the grill to medium-high heat. Proceed to season the chicken breasts thoroughly with salt and pepper.

Grill the chicken breasts for 6-8 minutes each side until they are completely done and no longer pink in the middle. Once done, take them from the grill and let them rest for a few minutes before slicing.

In a generously-sized salad bowl, add the mixed greens, sliced cucumber, cherry tomatoes, sliced red onion, and black olives.

In a separate small bowl, mix together the olive oil, red wine vinegar, Dijon mustard, salt, and pepper to produce the delicious vinaigrette.

Add the sliced grilled chicken to the salad dish. Drizzle the prepared olive oil vinaigrette over the salad and carefully mix everything together to get an equal coverage of the dressing.

Night Prepared Oats

Serving	Kcal	Carbs	Proteins	Fats	Fiber
1	250	40g	8g	7g	9g

Prep Time: 5 minutes
Total Time: Overnight (at least 4 hours)

Ingredients

- 1/2 cup rolled oats
- 1 tablespoon chia seeds
- 1/2 cup unsweetened almond milk
- 1/4 teaspoon vanilla extract
- 1/2 cup strawberries, blueberries, raspberries
- 1 tablespoon maple syrup
- Sliced almonds, coconut flakes

Step by Step Preparations

Start by combining your components in a mason jar or airtight container. Combine the rolled oats, chia seeds, almond milk, and vanilla essence, ensuring thorough mixing.

Gently combine the mixed berries and maple syrup, spreading them evenly throughout the mixture. Seal the jar or container with a lid and refrigerate overnight or for a minimum of 4 hours, enabling the oats and chia seeds to absorb the liquid and soften.

.When ready to serve, give the oats a slight toss. If the consistency is too thick for your taste, add a splash of extra almond milk until you get your ideal texture. Finish by topping your overnight oats with sliced almonds and coconut flakes

Turkey and avocado lettuce wraps

Serving	Kcal	Carbs	Proteins	Fats	Fiber
4	250	10g	20g	15g	5g

Prep Time: 15 minutes
Cooking Time: 10 minutes
Total Time: 25 minutes

Ingredients

- 1 lb ground turkey
- 1 ripe avocado, peeled, pitted, and sliced
- 1 head iceberg or butter lettuce, leaves separated
- 1 bell pepper, thinly sliced
- 1 tablespoon olive oil
- 1 teaspoon ground cumin
- 1 teaspoon paprika
- 1/2 teaspoon garlic powder
- Salt and pepper

Step by Step Preparations

Begin by heating olive oil in a pan over medium heat. Introduce the ground turkey, using a spoon to break it up while it cooks. Allow it to brown and cook through, normally taking around 5-7 minutes.

Season the turkey with ground cumin, paprika, garlic powder, salt, and pepper. Stir the spices into the turkey, ensuring uniform distribution, and cook for a further 1-2 minutes. Once done, take the skillet from heat and put it aside.

On a serving tray, arrange lettuce leaves in an attractive way. Spoon a good piece of the cooked turkey onto each lettuce leaf. Top the turkey with sliced avocado and strips of bell pepper

Smoothie and protein powder

Serving	Kcal	Carbs	Proteins	Fats	Fiber
1	250	35g	20g	5g	7g

Prep Time: 5 minutes
Cooking Time: 0 min.
Total Time: 5 minutes

Ingredients

- 1 ripe banana, peeled and sliced
- 1 cup fresh spinach leaves
- 1 cup unsweetened almond milk
- 1 scoop unflavored or protein powder
- Ice cubes

Step by Step Preparations

Start by combining the sliced banana, fresh spinach leaves, almond milk, and protein powder in a blender. For a colder, denser texture, perhaps put a handful of ice cubes in the blender.

Blend the ingredients on high speed until they form a smooth, creamy consistency, often approximately 1-2 minutes. Be careful to scrape down the edges of the blender as required throughout the blending operation.

Once mixed, taste the smoothie and fine-tune the sweetness or thickness by introducing extra banana or almond milk

Quinoa salad with chickpeas

Serving	Kcal	Carbs	Proteins	Fats	Fiber
4	320	45g	12g	11g	7g

Prep Time: 15 minutes
Cooking Time: 15 minutes
Total Time: 30 minutes

Ingredients

- 1 cup quinoa, rinsed
- 2 cups water or vegetable broth
- 1 can (15 oz) chickpeas, drained and rinsed
- 1 cup cherry tomatoes, halved
- 1/4 cup fresh parsley, chopped
- 1/4 cup fresh cilantro, chopped
- Lemon-Tahini Dressing:
- 1/4 cup tahini
- 2 tablespoons lemon juice
- 2 tablespoons water
- 1 clove garlic, minced
- Salt and pepper

Step by Step Preparations

Start by boiling water or vegetable broth in a medium pot until it reaches a boil. Add the quinoa, then reduce the heat to a simmer, covering the pot, and cook for 15 minutes or until the quinoa is soft and has absorbed the water.

Once done, remove the pot from heat and allow the quinoa to cool slightly. In a wide mixing basin, combine the cooked quinoa with chickpeas, cherry tomatoes, parsley, and cilantro.

In a separate small bowl, mix together tahini, lemon juice, water, minced garlic, salt, and pepper until a smooth, creamy consistency is obtained.

Pour the lemon-tahini dressing over the quinoa and vegetable combination, gently tossing until everything is uniformly covered. Lastly, taste the food and adjust spice

Greek yogurt parfait with berries

Serving	Kcal	Carbs	Proteins	Fats	Fiber
1	250	25g	15g	5g	3g

Prep Time: 5 minutes
Total Time: 5 minutes

Ingredients

1/2 cup plain Greek yogurt

1/4 cup strawberries, blueberries, raspberries

2 tablespoons gluten-free granola

Honey or maple syrup, fresh mint leaves

Step by Step Preparations

Start by stacking half of the Greek yogurt in a serving glass or dish. Top the yogurt layer with half of the mixed berries. Sprinkle half of the gluten-free granola over the berries.

Repeat the layers, using the remaining Greek yogurt, berries, and granola. For extra sweetness, sprinkle honey or maple syrup over the top to your preference. Finish by garnishing with fresh mint leaves to offer a splash of color and additional freshness.

Turkey and vegetable soup

Serving	Kcal	Carbs	Proteins	Fats	Fiber
4	250	15g	20g	12g	4g

Prep Time: 15 minutes
Cooking Time: 30 minutes
Total Time: 45 minutes

Ingredients

- 1 lb ground turkey
- 4 cups chicken or vegetable broth
- 2 carrots, diced
- 2 stalks celery, diced
- 1 cup spinach, chopped
- 1 small zucchini, diced
- 1/2 cup gluten-free crackers, crushed
- 1 tablespoon olive oil
- 1 teaspoon dried thyme
- Salt and pepper

Step by Step Preparations

Start by heating olive oil in a big saucepan over medium heat. Add the ground turkey and heat until it's browned, using a spoon to break it into little pieces, which should take roughly 5-7 minutes.

Incorporate the diced carrots and celery into the saucepan, simmering for a further 3-4 minutes until they begin to soften slightly. Once melted, add in the chicken or vegetable broth, bringing the mixture to a slow boil.

Add the diced zucchini and dried thyme to the saucepan, continuing to boil for another 10-15 minutes until the veggies achieve a soft consistency.

Introduce the chopped spinach into the saucepan, letting it simmer for a further 2-3 minutes until it wilts. Season the soup with salt and pepper according to your taste preferences.

When ready to serve, pour the soup into serving dishes and top each bowl with a tablespoon of mashed gluten-free crackers

Omelet with mushrooms

Serving	Kcal	Carbs	Proteins	Fats	Fiber
2	250	6g	15g	18g	2g

Prep Time: 10 minutes
Cooking Time: 10 minutes
Total Time: 20 minutes

Ingredients

- 4 large eggs
- 1 cup mushrooms, sliced
- 1 cup spinach, chopped
- 1/4 cup almond or soy-based cheese, grated
- 1 tablespoon olive oil
- Salt and pepper

Step by Step Preparations

In a medium-sized mixing basin, carefully break the eggs and whisk them with a fork or whisk until softly beaten. Season with salt and pepper according to taste.

Warm the olive oil in a non-stick skillet over medium heat. Add the sliced mushrooms and sauté for 3-4 minutes until they begin to soften.

Introduce the chopped spinach to the pan and continue cooking for another 2-3 minutes until it wilts. Carefully pour the beaten eggs over the mushrooms and spinach in the skillet, turning the pan to achieve uniform distribution.

Allow the omelet to cook undisturbed for 2-3 minutes until the edges start to firm. Evenly sprinkle the shredded dairy-free cheese over one side of the omelet.

Using a spatula, carefully fold the second half of the omelet over the cheese-covered half. Continue cooking for another 2-3 minutes until the cheese melts and the omelet is thoroughly cooked through.

Quinoa and black bean salad

Serving	Kcal	Carbs	Proteins	Fats	Fiber
4	350	45g	11g	15g	10g

Prep Time: 15 minutes
Cooking Time: 15 minutes
Total Time: 30 minutes

Ingredients

- 1 cup quinoa, rinsed
- 2 cups water or vegetable broth
- 1 can (15 oz) black beans, drained and rinsed
- 1 cup frozen corn kernels, thawed
- 1 avocado, diced
- 1/4 cup fresh cilantro, chopped
- 1 green onion, thinly sliced

Lime Dressing

- 2 tablespoons olive oil
- 2 tablespoons lime juice
- 1 teaspoon maple syrup or honey
- 1/2 teaspoon ground cumin
- Salt and pepper

Step by Step Preparations

Begin by boiling the quinoa as per the directions on the box, using either water or low FODMAP vegetable broth for added taste. Once cooked, use a fork to fluff the quinoa and let it cool to room temperature.

In a big mixing dish, add the cooked quinoa, black beans, thawed corn kernels, diced avocado, chopped cilantro, and sliced green onion.

In a second small bowl, mix together the olive oil, lime juice, and maple syrup or honey, along with ground cumin, salt, and pepper to make the lime dressing.

Carefully pour the lime dressing over the quinoa and black bean combination, ensuring complete covering by gently tossing everything together.

Taste the food and adjust spices if required. Serve immediately for rapid pleasure, or chill for at least 30 minutes

Smoothie bowl and pumpkin seeds

Serving	Kcal	Carbs	Proteins	Fats	Fiber
1	300	40g	7g	14g	7g

Prep Time: 5 minutes
Total Time: 10 minutes

Ingredients

1 ripe banana, frozen

1/2 cup strawberries or blueberries

1/2 cup lactose-free yogurt or almond or coconut

1/4 cup granola

1 tablespoon shredded coconut

1 tablespoon pumpkin seeds

Step by Step Preparations

Start by pouring the frozen banana, berries, and yogurt into a blender. Blend the ingredients until they attain a smooth and creamy consistency. Transfer the smoothie into a bowl. Finish off by topping the smoothie with sliced banana, shredded coconut, pumpkin seeds, and granola.

Chicken with tamari sauce

Serving	Kcal	Carbs	Proteins	Fats	Fiber
4	200	10g	20g	8g	3g

Prep Time: 15 minutes
Cooking Time: 15 minutes
Total Time: 30 minutes

Ingredients

2 boneless, skinless chicken breasts, thinly sliced

2 cups bell peppers, broccoli, and snap peas, sliced

2 cloves garlic, minced

1 tablespoon ginger, minced

3 tablespoons tamari sauce

2 tablespoons olive oil

4 cups cooked brown rice

Step by Step Preparations

Start by heating 1 tablespoon of olive oil in a large pan or wok over medium-high heat. Add the cut chicken breasts and heat them until they attain a browned, well cooked consistency, normally taking approximately 5-7 minutes.

Once done, take the chicken from the pan and put it aside shortly. In the same skillet, insert the remaining tablespoon of olive oil. Incorporate the minced garlic and ginger, letting them to fry for 1 minute until they unleash their delicious scent.

Next, add the sliced mixed veggies to the pan and stir-fry them for roughly 5 minutes until they achieve a tender-crisp stage. Reintroduce the cooked chicken to the pan with the veggies.

Pour the tamari sauce over the chicken and veggies, ensuring full covering by tossing everything together. Cook the mixture for a further 2-3 minutes, stirring regularly to properly spread the flavors. Finally, serve the chicken and vegetable stir-fry hot over cooked brown rice

Chia seed pudding with berries

Serving	Kcal	Carbs	Proteins	Fats	Fiber
2	150	20g	4g	7g	9g

Prep Time: 5 minutes
Cooking Time: 0
Total Time: 5 minutes

Ingredients

1/4 cup chia seeds

1 cup unsweetened almond milk

1 tablespoon maple syrup

1/2 teaspoon vanilla extract

1 cup strawberries, blueberries, and raspberries

Step By Step Preparations

Start by grabbing a mixing bowl or container. In it, add the chia seeds, almond milk, maple syrup (if selecting for sweetness), and vanilla essence. Thoroughly whisk the mixture to ensure all components are properly incorporated.

Once blended, cover the bowl or jar and store it in the refrigerator overnight, or for a minimum of 4 hours. This causes the chia seeds to soak up the liquid and turn into a pudding-like consistency.

When ready to serve, give the chia pudding a thorough toss to uniformly disperse the seeds and avoid any clumps from developing.

Divide the prepared chia pudding into serving dishes or glasses. To end, liberally top each serving with a choice of mixed berries

Lentil and vegetable soup

Serving	Kcal	Carbs	Proteins	Fats	Fiber
4	200	30g	10g	5g	10g

Prep Time: 15 minutes
Cooking Time: 35 minutes
Total Time: 50 minutes

Ingredients

- 1 cup dry green or brown lentils, rinsed and drained
- 4 cups vegetable broth
- 2 carrots, diced
- 2 stalks celery, diced
- 1 cup spinach, chopped
- 1 onion, diced
- 2 cloves garlic, minced
- 2 tablespoons olive oil
- 1 teaspoon dried thyme
- Salt and pepper
- Gluten-free bread slices

Step by Step Preparations

Start by heating the olive oil in a big saucepan over medium heat. Introduce the chopped onion to the saucepan and simmer until it becomes transparent, 3-4 minutes.

Afterward, add the minced garlic to the saucepan and simmer for a further 1-2 minutes until its scent becomes aromatic.

Incorporate the chopped carrots and celery into the saucepan, simmering them for around 5 minutes until they slightly soften.

Season the mixture by tossing in the dried thyme, salt, and pepper. Proceed to add the washed lentils and veggie broth to the pot. Bring the soup to a boil, then decrease the heat to low, cover, and allow it to simmer for 20-25 minutes, or until the lentils acquire softness.

Once the lentils are cooked, add the chopped spinach to the saucepan and stir until it wilts, 2-3 minutes. Taste the soup and adjust the seasoning if required by adding additional salt and pepper to suit your palate. Serve the hot soup with pieces of gluten-free bread

IBS friendly Dinner Options

Baked salmon and quinoa

Serving	Kcal	Carbs	Proteins	Fats	Fiber
4	400	25g	30g	20g	5g

Prep Time: 15 minutes
Cooking Time: 25 minutes
Total Time: 40 minutes

Ingredients

- 4 salmon filets (about 4-6 oz each), skin removed
- 1 cup quinoa, rinsed
- 2 cups water vegetable broth
- 4 large carrots, peeled and cut into sticks
- 2 tablespoons olive oil
- 1 teaspoon dried dill (or 2 teaspoons fresh dill), chopped
- 1 teaspoon paprika
- Salt and pepper

Step by Step Preparations

To begin, preheat your oven to 400°F (200°C) and line a baking sheet with parchment paper. In a medium saucepan, bring either water or vegetable broth to a boil. Add the rinsed quinoa, then decrease the heat to low, cover, and let it simmer for 15 minutes or until the quinoa is cooked and the liquid is absorbed.

Once done, take it from the heat and let it remain covered for 5 minutes before fluffing it with a fork. While the quinoa is cooking, cover the carrot sticks with 1 tablespoon of olive oil, dried dill, paprika, salt, and pepper on the prepared baking sheet, ensuring they're spread out evenly in a single layer.

Transfer the baking sheet to the preheated oven and roast the carrots for 20-25 minutes, or until they are soft and acquire a mild caramelization, remembering to toss them halfway during the cooking procedure.

As the carrots roast, prepare the salmon by rubbing the filets with the remaining olive oil and seasoning them with salt and pepper according to your desire.

After the carrots have roasted for 10 minutes, add the seasoned salmon filets to the baking sheet, laying them skin-side down.

Return the baking pan to the oven and continue baking for another 10-15 minutes, or until the salmon is thoroughly cooked and flakes easily with a fork. To serve, place the baked salmon and roasted carrots on a bed of cooked quinoa

Stir-fried tofu and brown rice

Serving	Kcal	Carbs	Proteins	Fats	Fiber
4	250	12g	15g	18g	4g

Prep Time: 15 minutes
Cooking Time: 15 minutes
Total Time: 30 minutes

Ingredients

- 1 block (14 oz) firm tofu, pressed and cubed
- 2 cups broccoli florets
- 1 bell pepper, thinly sliced
- 2 cloves garlic, minced
- 1 tablespoon ginger, minced
- 2 tablespoons low-sodium soy sauce
- 1 tablespoon sesame oil
- 2 tablespoons olive or canola oil
- Cooked brown rice

Step by Step Preparations

To start, cover the tofu block in paper towels or a clean kitchen towel, then exert pressure with a heavy item, such as a cast iron pan or a few cans, to drain excess water. Allow it to press for 15 minutes.

While the tofu is pressing, prepare the veggies accordingly: chop the broccoli into tiny florets, finely slice the bell pepper, and mince both the garlic and ginger.

In a large skillet or wok, heat 1 tablespoon of vegetable oil over medium-high heat. Once heated, add the cubed tofu to the pan in a single layer. Cook for approximately 5-7 minutes, rotating regularly, until all sides attain a golden brown, crispy texture.

Once done, take the tofu from the pan and put it aside.
In the same skillet, combine the remaining tablespoon of vegetable oil. Add the minced garlic and ginger, letting them simmer for 1 minute until fragrant.

Add the broccoli florets and sliced bell pepper to the pan, stirring periodically. Stir-fry the veggies for approximately 3-4 minutes, or until they attain a soft but crunchy consistency.

Add the cooked tofu and veggies back to the pan. Drizzle the mixture with low-sodium soy sauce and sesame oil. Stir-fry for a further 2-3 minutes until everything is cooked through and thoroughly mixed. Serve hot over cooked brown rice for a great supper.

Grilled shrimp skewers and marinara sauce

Serving	Kcal	Carbs	Proteins	Fats	Fiber
4	250	12g	25g	12g	5g

Prep Time: 20 minutes
Cooking Time: 10 minutes
Total Time: 30 minutes

For the Grilled Shrimp

- 1 pound large shrimp, peeled and deveined
- 2 tablespoons olive oil
- 2 cloves garlic, minced
- 1 tablespoon lemon juice
- Salt and pepper

For the Zucchini Noodles

- 4 medium zucchinis, spiralized into noodles
- 1 tablespoon olive oil
- Salt and pepper

For the Marinara Sauce

- 1 can (14 oz) diced tomatoes
- 2 cloves garlic, minced
- 1 teaspoon dried oregano
- 1 teaspoon dried basil
- Salt and pepper

Step by Step Preparations

Begin by mixing the shrimp with olive oil, chopped garlic, lemon juice, salt, and pepper in a bowl, ensuring uniform covering. Skewer the seasoned shrimp on skewers.

Preheat a grill or grill pan over medium-high heat. Grill the shrimp skewers for 2-3 minutes each side, until they become pink and cook through. Once done, put them aside.

In a large pan over medium heat, heat olive oil. Add the zucchini noodles and sauté for 3-4 minutes until soft but slightly crunchy. Season with salt and pepper to taste, then remove from fire and put aside.

In the same pan used for the zucchini noodles, sauté minced garlic for 1 minute until fragrant. Incorporate chopped tomatoes, dried oregano, dry basil, salt, and pepper into the skillet. Stir well to mix.

Simmer the sauce for 5-7 minutes, stirring periodically, until it thickens slightly. Adjust seasoning as required. Divide the zucchini noodles among serving dishes. Top the zucchini noodles with grilled shrimp skewers.

Spoon marinara sauce liberally over the shrimp and pasta. Finish by garnishing with fresh basil leaves.

Baked chicken breast and mashed sweet potatoes

Serving	Kcal	Carbs	Proteins	Fats	Fiber
4	350	30g	30g	12g	7g

Prep Time: 15 minutes
Cooking Time: 45 minutes
Total Time: 1 hour

Ingredients

- 4 boneless, skinless chicken breasts
- 1 pound green beans, trimmed
- 4 medium sweet potatoes, peeled and diced
- 2 tablespoons olive oil
- 1 teaspoon garlic powder
- 1 teaspoon paprika
- Salt and pepper

Step by Step Preparations

Start by preheating your oven to 400°F (200°C). Begin by putting the diced sweet potatoes in a saucepan of boiling water, letting them simmer until soft, 15-20 minutes. Once tender, rinse the sweet potatoes and put them aside.

While the sweet potatoes are cooking, concentrate on preparing the chicken breasts. Arrange them on a baking sheet lined with parchment paper. Drizzle the chicken breasts with olive oil and sprinkle them with garlic powder, paprika, salt, and pepper.

Place the seasoned chicken breasts in the preheated oven and bake for 20-25 minutes, or until they acquire an internal temperature of 165°F (75°C) and are well cooked.

Meanwhile, steam the green beans until they achieve a soft consistency, normally taking approximately 5-7 minutes. You may employ a steamer basket or just boil them in a saucepan with a tiny bit of water.

Once the sweet potatoes are cooked, continue to mash them using a potato masher or fork until they acquire a smooth texture. Season the mashed sweet potatoes with salt and pepper to taste. To serve, put the roasted chicken breasts beside the steaming green beans and mashed sweet potatoes

Grilled steak with roasted asparagus

Serving	Kcal	Carbs	Proteins	Fats	Fiber
4	400	25g	25g	20g	4g

Prep Time: 15 minutes
Marinating Time: 30 minutes
Cooking Time: 20 minutes
Total Time: 65 minutes

Ingredients

- 4 small sirloin steaks (about 4-6 oz each)
- 1 bunch asparagus, trimmed
- 1 cup quinoa, rinsed
- 2 cups vegetable broth
- 2 tablespoons olive oil
- 2 tablespoons balsamic vinegar
- 2 cloves garlic, minced
- 1 teaspoon dried thyme
- Salt and pepper

Step by Step Preparations

If picking to marinate the steak, begin by putting the steaks in a shallow dish. Season them liberally with salt, pepper, chopped garlic, dried thyme, olive oil, and balsamic vinegar.

Cover the dish and refrigerate for a minimum of 30 minutes, allowing the flavors to penetrate, or marinate for up to 4 hours for increased taste.

Preheat the grill to medium-high heat. Remove the steaks from the marinade, discarding any extra liquid. Grill the steaks for 4-6 minutes each side, or until they achieve the desired amount of doneness.

Once done, take them from the grill and let them rest for 5 minutes to enable the juices to redistribute before serving. Meanwhile, while the steaks are cooking, prepare the oven to 400°F (200°C).

Arrange the trimmed asparagus stalks on a baking sheet, sprinkle them with olive oil, and season with salt and pepper. Roast the asparagus in the oven for 10-12 minutes, ensuring they are soft but maintain a crisp texture.

In a medium saucepan, bring the vegetable broth to a boil. Add the rinsed quinoa, then decrease the heat to low, cover, and let it simmer for 15-20 minutes, or until the quinoa is cooked and the liquid is absorbed.

Fluff the quinoa with a fork to separate the grains. To serve, offer the grilled steak with the roasted asparagus and quinoa pilaf

Baked cod and wild rice

Serving	Kcal	Carbs	Proteins	Fats	Fiber
4	350	30g	30g	13g	7g

Prep Time: 15 minutes
Cooking Time: 25 minutes
Total Time: 40 minutes

Ingredients

- 4 cod filets (about 6 oz each)
- 1 lb Brussels sprouts, trimmed and halved
- 1 cup wild rice
- 2 tablespoons olive oil
- 2 cloves garlic, minced
- 1 teaspoon dried thyme
- Salt and pepper

Step by Step Preparations

Start by preheating the oven to 400°F (200°C) and line a baking sheet with parchment paper or aluminum foil. In a small bowl, add the minced garlic, dried thyme, salt, and pepper.

Lay the fish filets on the prepared baking sheet. Brush each filet with olive oil and sprinkle the garlic and thyme mixture over them.

Arrange the halved Brussels sprouts around the fish filets on the baking sheet. Drizzle them with olive oil and season with salt and pepper.

Roast everything in the preheated oven for 20-25 minutes, or until the cod is well cooked and readily flakes with a fork, and the Brussels sprouts reach a golden brown, soft texture.

While the cod and Brussels sprouts are baking, cook the wild rice according to the package directions until it's soft and fluffy. Once everything is cooked to perfection, divide the wild rice, roasted Brussels sprouts, and baked fish among serving dishes.

Turkey meatballs and marinara sauce

Serving	Kcal	Carbs	Proteins	Fats	Fiber
4	300	20g	25g	15g	5g

Prep Time: 20 minutes
Cooking Time: 40 minutes
Total Time: 1 hour

Ingredients

- 1 medium spaghetti squash
- 1 pound ground turkey
- 1 egg
- 1/4 cup gluten-free breadcrumbs
- 2 tablespoons fresh parsley, chopped
- 1 teaspoon dried oregano
- 1/2 teaspoon garlic powder
- Salt and pepper
- 2 cups marinara sauce

Step by Step Preparations

Start by preheating your oven to 400°F (200°C). Proceed to split the spaghetti squash lengthwise and remove the seeds. Place the squash halves, with the sliced side down, onto a parchment paper-lined baking sheet. Bake them for 35-40 minutes, or until the squash becomes soft and can be easily punctured with a fork.

Once roasted, take the squash out of the oven and allow it to cool somewhat. While the squash is baking, make the turkey meatballs. In a large mixing bowl, combine the ground turkey, egg, gluten-free breadcrumbs, chopped parsley, dried oregano, garlic powder, salt, and pepper. Thoroughly mix the ingredients until they are fully blended.

Shape the turkey mixture into meatballs, aiming for a diameter of approximately 1 inch. Heat a non-stick skillet over medium heat. Add the meatballs to the pan and cook them for 8-10 minutes, flipping them regularly, until they acquire a golden brown color on both sides and are cooked through.

In a separate saucepan, cook the marinara sauce over medium heat until it is heated through. Once the spaghetti squash has cooled down enough to handle, use a fork to scrape the flesh into strands.

To serve, split the spaghetti squash equally among plates, top it with the turkey meatballs, then liberally ladle the marinara sauce over the meatballs.

IBS Friendly Desserts and Sweet Treats

IBS Fruit Salad

Serving	Kcal	Carbs	Proteins	Fats	Fiber
4	60	15g	1g	0	2g

Prep Time: 15 minutes
Cooking Time: 0 min.
Total Time: 15 minutes

Ingredients

- 2 cups strawberries, blueberries, pineapple, grapes, and kiwi, diced
- 1 tablespoon fresh lemon juice
- 1 tablespoon maple syrup or honey
- Fresh mint leaves

Step by Step Preparations

Start by cleaning and prepping the fruits as required. Dice bigger fruits such as pineapple and kiwi into bite-sized pieces. In a big mixing basin, put together the choice of fruits.

Drizzle the freshly squeezed lemon juice over the fruits. For those desiring a bit of sweetness, maple syrup or honey can be used.

With a soft hand, toss the fruits until they are well covered with the lemon juice and preferred sweetener. Transfer the colorful fruit salad to a serving bowl or divide among individual serving plates. For a finishing touch, garnish the dish with sprigs of fresh mint leaves.

Dark Chocolate

Serving	Kcal	Carbs	Proteins	Fats	Fiber
8	120	8g	2g	11g	3g

Prep Time: 10 minutes
Cooking Time: 0 min.
Total Time: 10 minutes

Ingredients

- 1 cup unsweetened cocoa powder
- 1/2 cup coconut oil, melted
- 1/4 cup maple syrup
- 1 teaspoon vanilla extract
- Pinch of salt

Step by Step Preparations

In a medium-sized dish, begin by sifting the cocoa powder to remove any lumps. Incorporate the melted coconut oil, maple syrup (if going for sweetness), vanilla essence, and a bit of salt into the cocoa powder.

Stir the amalgamation until it gets a smooth and homogenous texture. Prepare a baking sheet or tray by lining it with parchment paper.

Transfer the chocolate mixture onto the prepared baking sheet, using a spatula to spread it out evenly to your desired thickness. Place the baking sheet in the refrigerator for 1-2 hours, enabling the chocolate to firm and set.

Once the chocolate has hardened, extract it from the refrigerator and break it into separate pieces. For storage, put the chocolate in an airtight container in the refrigerator, where it may preserve its freshness for up to two weeks.

Banana Nice Cream

Serving	Kcal	Carbs	Proteins	Fats	Fiber
2	100	25g	1g	0.5g	3g

Prep Time: 5 minutes
Freezing Time: 4 hours
Total Time: 4 hours 5 minutes

Ingredients

- 2 ripe bananas, peeled and sliced
- 1/4 cup unsweetened almond milk
- 1 teaspoon pure vanilla extract
- Chopped nuts, shredded coconut, or dark chocolate chips.

Step by Step Preparations

Begin by putting the sliced bananas on a baking sheet lined with parchment paper, ensuring they are in a single layer. Freeze the bananas for a minimum of 4 hours or overnight until they are totally frozen.

After the bananas have frozen, add them to either a food processor or a high-speed blender. Into the blender, pour the unsweetened almond milk and add the pure vanilla extract.

Blend the ingredients until they achieve a smooth and creamy consistency, being careful to scrape down the edges of the blender or food processor as required. The resultant combination should mirror the texture of soft serve ice cream.

For extra taste and texture, put any combination of chopped nuts, shredded coconut, or dark chocolate chips into the recipe.

Oatmeal Cookies

Serving	Kcal	Carbs	Proteins	Fats	Fiber
12	100	12g	1.5g	5g	1.5g

Prep Time: 10 minutes
Cooking Time: 12 minutes
Total Time: 22 minutes

Ingredients

- 1 cup rolled oats
- 1/2 cup oat flour
- 1/4 cup coconut oil, melted
- 1/4 cup pure maple syrup or honey
- 1/4 cup unsweetened applesauce
- 1 teaspoon vanilla extract
- 1/2 teaspoon ground cinnamon
- 1/4 teaspoon salt
- 1/4 cup raisins or chopped dried cranberries

Step by Step Preparations

2Start by preheating your oven to 350°F (175°C) and line a baking sheet with parchment paper. In a substantially sized mixing basin, combine the rolled oats, oat flour, cinnamon, and salt.

In a separate dish, mix together the melted coconut oil, maple syrup or honey, unsweetened applesauce, and vanilla extract until fully incorporated.

Combine the wet components with the dry ones, mixing until a homogeneous consistency emerges. If desired, carefully mix in the raisins or chopped dried cranberries.

Using a spoon or cookie scoop, put spoonfuls of dough onto the prepared baking sheet, ensuring they are spaced approximately 2 inches apart. Gently flatten each cookie gently using your fingertips or the back of a spoon.

Place the baking sheet in the preheated oven and bake for 10-12 minutes, or until the edges of the cookies become golden brown.

Once cooked, remove the cookies from the oven and allow them to cool on the baking sheet for 5 minutes. Afterward, move them to a wire rack to cool fully.

Coconut Yogurt Parfait

Serving	Kcal	Carbs	Proteins	Fats	Fiber
1	300	25g	6g	20g	5g

Prep Time: 10 minutes
Total Time: 10 minutes

Ingredients

- 1/2 cup lactose-free coconut yogurt
- 1/4 cup granola
- 1/4 cup fresh strawberries, sliced
- 1 tablespoon shredded coconut (unsweetened)
- 1 tablespoon almonds or walnuts

Step by Step Preparations

Begin by preparing a glass or serving basin for layering.
Start the layering procedure by laying a foundation of lactose-free coconut yogurt at the bottom of the bowl.

On top of the yogurt, put a thick coating of low FODMAP granola. Proceed to spread a layer of cut strawberries over the granola, ensuring uniform distribution.

Sprinkle shredded coconut and chopped almonds on top of the strawberries, providing a delicious crunchy taste

Repeat the stacking technique until all the components are used up, ensuring each layer is equally spread. Conclude the layers with a last sprinkling of shredded coconut and chopped nuts on top

Rice Pudding

Serving	Kcal	Carbs	Proteins	Fats	Fiber
4	180	30g	5g	4g	1g

Prep Time: 5 minutes
Cooking Time: 30 minutes
Total Time: 35 minutes

Ingredients

- 1/2 cup Arborio rice or short-grain white rice
- 2 cups lactose-free milk or unsweetened almond milk
- 1/4 cup maple syrup or sugar
- 1 teaspoon vanilla extract
- 1/2 teaspoon ground cinnamon
- Pinch of salt

Step by Step Preparations

In a medium saucepan, mix the rice, lactose-free milk, optional maple syrup, vanilla essence, ground cinnamon, and a sprinkle of salt.

Bring the mixture to a moderate boil over medium heat, then decrease the heat to low and simmer uncovered, stirring periodically, for 25-30 minutes or until the rice acquires a soft texture and the pudding thickens to your preference.

Should the pudding thicken too much, just add a touch more milk to adapt to your chosen consistency.

Once the rice is cooked through and the pudding has achieved the required thickness, take the pot from the heat and allow it to cool slightly before serving.

Peanut Butter Energy Balls

Serving	Kcal	Carbs	Proteins	Fats	Fiber
12	120	12g	4g	7g	2g

Prep Time: 15 minutes
Cooking Time: 0 min.
Total Time: 15 minutes

Ingredients

- 1 cup rolled oats
- 1/2 cup smooth peanut butter (unsweetened and no added oils)
- 1/4 cup maple syrup or honey
- 1/4 cup unsweetened shredded coconut
- 2 tablespoons ground flaxseed
- 1 teaspoon vanilla extract
- Pinch of salt
- Dark chocolate chips, chopped nuts, dried fruit

Step by Step Preparations

In a large mixing basin, assemble the rolled oats, peanut butter, maple syrup or honey, shredded coconut, ground flaxseed, vanilla essence, and a sprinkle of salt if preferred.

Thoroughly mix all the ingredients until they are equally incorporated. Should the mixture look too dry, try introducing a touch more peanut butter or maple syrup to boost cohesiveness.

For extra taste and texture, integrate optional add-ins such dark chocolate chips, chopped almonds, or dried fruit. Ensure these ingredients are uniformly disseminated throughout the mixture.

Once the mixture gets a consistent consistency, shape tiny amounts into bite-sized balls, 1 inch in diameter, using your hands.

Arrange the created energy balls on a baking sheet coated with parchment paper, then refrigerate them for at least 30 minutes to aid stiffness.

After cooling, place the energy balls into an airtight container and keep them in the refrigerator until you're ready to indulge in these healthy delights.

(use maple syrup for a vegan option)

Baked Apples

Serving	Kcal	Carbs	Proteins	Sugar	Fiber
4	90	24g	0	19g	4g

Prep Time: 10 minutes
Cooking Time: 30 minutes
Total Time: 40 minutes

Ingredients

- 4 medium-sized apples, Granny Smith or Honeycrisp
- 2 tablespoons maple syrup or honey
- 1 teaspoon ground cinnamon
- 1/4 cup chopped walnuts or pecans
- 1 tablespoon melted coconut oil or butter
- Pinch of salt

Step by Step Preparations

Start by preheating your oven to 375°F (190°C). Prepare a baking dish by coating it with parchment paper or gently greasing it with coconut oil or butter.

After washing the apples, gently remove the cores using an apple corer or a tiny knife, being sure to keep the bottoms intact. Arrange the prepped apples in the baking dish.

In a small bowl, mix the maple syrup or honey, ground cinnamon, chopped almonds, melted coconut oil or butter, and a sprinkle of salt.

Carefully pour the cinnamon mixture into the middle of each apple, ensuring the holes are uniformly filled.

Place the baking dish with the filled apples in the preheated oven and bake for 25-30 minutes, or until the apples are soft and the filling is bubbling.

Almond Flour Blueberry Muffins

Serving	Kcal	Carbs	Proteins	Fats	Fiber
12	180	10g	5g	14g	3g

Prep Time: 10 minutes
Cooking Time: 25 minutes
Total Time: 35 minutes

Ingredients:

- 2 cups almond flour
- 1/4 cup coconut flour
- 1/4 cup maple syrup or honey
- 3 large eggs
- 1/4 cup coconut oil, melted
- 1 teaspoon vanilla extract
- 1 teaspoon baking powder
- 1/4 teaspoon salt
- 1 cup fresh blueberries

Step by Step Preparations

To start, preheat your oven to 350°F (175°C) and prepare your muffin pan by filling it with paper liners or greasing the muffin cups with coconut oil.

In a big mixing basin, add the almond flour, coconut flour, baking powder, and salt, ensuring thorough mixing. In a separate dish, mix together the eggs, melted coconut oil, and maple syrup or honey, along with the vanilla essence.

Pour the wet components into the dry ingredients, mixing until barely incorporated, being mindful not to overmix the batter. Gently fold in the blueberries until they are uniformly distributed throughout the batter.

Divide the batter equally among the muffin cups, filling each 2/3 full. Place the muffin tray in the preheated oven and bake for 20-25 minutes, or until the tops become golden brown and a toothpick inserted into the middle of a muffin comes out clean.

Once cooked, allow the muffins to rest in the tray for 5 minutes before transferring them to a wire rack to cool entirely.

References

Algera, J. P., Colomier, E., & Simrén, M. (2019). The Dietary Management of Patients with Irritable Bowel Syndrome: A Narrative Review of the Existing and Emerging Evidence. *Nutrients*, *11*(9), 2162. https://doi.org/10.3390/nu11092162

Ali, A., Weiss, T. R., McKee, D., Scherban, A., Khan, S., Fields, M., Apollo, D., & Mehal, W. Z. (2017). Efficacy of individualized diets in patients with irritable bowel syndrome: a randomized controlled trial. *BMJ Open Gastroenterology*, *4*(1), e000164. https://doi.org/10.1136/bmjgast-2017-000164

Chey, W. D. (2019). Elimination diets for irritable bowel Syndrome: Approaching the end of the beginning. *The American Journal of Gastroenterology*, *114*(2), 201–203. https://doi.org/10.14309/ajg.0000000000000099

Clinic, C. (2024, March 19). *Understanding the differences between IBD and IBS*. Cleveland Clinic. https://health.clevelandclinic.org/ibd-vs-ibs

Definition & Facts for Irritable Bowel Syndrome. (2022, July 23). National Institute of Diabetes and Digestive and Kidney Diseases. https://www.niddk.nih.gov/health-information/digestive-diseases/irritable-bowel-syndrome/definition-facts

Drisko, J., Bischoff, B., Hall, M., & McCallum, R. W. (2003). TREATING IRRITABLE BOWEL SYNDROME WITH a FOOD ELIMINATION DIET FOLLOWED BY FOOD CHALLENGE AND PROBIOTICS. *The American Journal of Gastroenterology*, *98*, S276. https://doi.org/10.1111/j.1572-0241.2003.08568.x

El-Salhy, M., Ystad, S., Mazzawi, T., & Gundersen, D. (2017). Dietary fiber in irritable bowel syndrome (Review). *International Journal of Molecular Medicine*, *40*(3), 607–613. https://doi.org/10.3892/ijmm.2017.3072

Foster, J. A., Rinaman, L., & Cryan, J. F. (2017). Stress & the gut-brain axis: Regulation by the microbiome. *Neurobiology of Stress*, 7, 124–136. https://doi.org/10.1016/j.ynstr.2017.03.001

Gastroadmin. (2018, September 25). *IBS Diet | Good Diet for IBS - London Gastroenterology Centre*. London Gastroenterology Centre. https://www.gastrolondon.co.uk/irritable-bowel-syndrome/diet-for-ibs/

Gastrocenternj. (2019, October 31). *Irritable bowel syndrome: symptoms and causes*. Gastro Center NJ. https://gastrocenternj.com/irritable-bowel-syndrome-symptoms-and-causes/

Gibson, P. R. (2017). History of the low FODMAP diet. *Journal of Gastroenterology and Hepatology*, *32*(S1), 5–7. https://doi.org/10.1111/jgh.13685

Irritable bowel Syndrome (IBS). (n.d.). Johns Hopkins Medicine. https://www.hopkinsmedicine.org/health/conditions-and-diseases/irritable-bowel-syndrome-ibs

Irritable Bowel Syndrome Studies | GI Motility and Neurogastroenterology | IU School of Medicine. (n.d.). https://medicine.iu.edu/internal-medicine/specialties/gastroenterology-hepatology/research/gi-motility/studies/irritable-bowel-syndrome

Jayasinghe, M., Karunanayake, V., Mohtashim, A., Caldera, D., Mendis, P., Prathiraja, O., Rashidi, F., & Damianos, J. (2024). The Role of Diet in the Management of Irritable Bowel Syndrome: A Comprehensive review. *Curēus.* https://doi.org/10.7759/cureus.54244

Large-scale genetic study reveals new clues for the shared origins of. (2021, November 5). University of Cambridge. https://www.cam.ac.uk/research/news/large-scale-genetic-study-reveals-new-clues-for-the-shared-origins-of-irritable-bowel-syndrome-and

Loosen, S. H., Kostev, K., Jördens, M. S., Luedde, T., & Roderburg, C. (2022). Overlap between irritable bowel syndrome and common gastrointestinal diagnoses: a retrospective cohort study of 29,553 outpatients in Germany. *BMC Gastroenterology*, *22*(1). https://doi.org/10.1186/s12876-022-02118-y

NHS inform. (2024, April 2). *Irritable bowel syndrome (IBS) | NHS inform*. NHS Inform. https://www.nhsinform.scot/illnesses-and-conditions/stomach-liver-and-gastrointestinal-tract/irritable-bowel-syndrome-ibs/

Raskov, H., Burcharth, J., Pommergaard, H., & Rosenberg, J. (2016). Irritable bowel syndrome, the microbiota and the gut-brain axis. *Gut Microbes*, *7*(5), 365–383. https://doi.org/10.1080/19490976.2016.1218585

Saha, L. (2014). Irritable bowel syndrome: Pathogenesis, diagnosis, treatment, and evidence-based medicine. *World Journal of Gastroenterology*, *20*(22), 6759. https://doi.org/10.3748/wjg.v20.i22.6759

Smith, E., Foxx–Orenstein, A. E., Marks, L., & Agrwal, N. (2020). Food sensitivity testing and elimination diets in the management of irritable bowel syndrome. *Journal of Osteopathic Medicine*, *120*(1), 19–23. https://doi.org/10.7556/jaoa.2020.008

Thomas, A., & Quigley, E. M. (2016). Dietary interventions and irritable bowel syndrome. In *Elsevier eBooks* (pp. 423–438). https://doi.org/10.1016/b978-0-12-802304-4.00020-7

Weaver, K. R., Melkus, G. D., & Henderson, W. A. (2017). Irritable bowel syndrome. *the American Journal of Nursing/American Journal of Nursing*, *117*(6), 48–55. https://doi.org/10.1097/01.naj.0000520253.57459.01

Website, N. (2023, September 11). *Irritable bowel syndrome (IBS)*. nhs.uk. https://www.nhs.uk/conditions/irritable-bowel-syndrome-ibs/

https://www.goodrx.com/health-topic/gastroenterology/ulcerative-colitis-ibs-crohns-differences

Appendices

Food Lists: High FODMAP Foods, Low FODMAP Foods

The following is a detailed list of high-FODMAPS foods organized by food groups:

Fruits

Apples

Cherries

Watermelon

Mangoes

Pears

Apricots

Plums

Nectarines

Peaches

Persimmons

Lychees

Rambutan

Blackberries

Boysenberries

Guava

Papaya

Vegetables

Onions

Garlic

Shallots

Leeks (white part)

Spring onions (white part)

Artichokes

Asparagus

Cauliflower

Mushrooms

Snow peas

Sugar snap peas

Savoy cabbage

Brussels sprouts

Beetroot

Celery

Sweet corn

Fennel

Okra

Legumes

Beans (kidney beans, black beans, pinto beans)

Lentils

Chickpeas

Split peas

Soybeans

Grains

Wheat-based products (bread, pasta, couscous)

Barley

Rye

Wheat-based cereals

Wheat-based baked goods (cakes, cookies, pastries)

Wheat-based snacks (crackers, pretzels)

Dairy Products

Milk

Soft cheese (ricotta, cottage cheese)

Ice cream

Custard

Yogurt with added inulin or high-FODMAP fruits

Sweeteners

Honey

Agave syrup

High-fructose corn syrup

Sorbitol

Mannitol

Xylitol

Isomalt

Miscellaneous

Applesauce

Fruit juice concentrate

Fruit jams and spreads containing high-FODMAP fruits

Sweetened condensed milk

Coconut water

Sodas and soft drinks sweetened with high-fructose corn syrup or polyols

Processed foods with added FODMAP-containing ingredients

Low FODMAP Pantry Staples:

- Gluten-Free Grains: Rice (white, brown, basmati), quinoa, certified gluten-free oats, cornmeal, and polenta.
- Low FODMAP Fruits and Vegetables: Strawberries, blueberries, raspberries, oranges, kiwi, grapes, spinach, lettuce, carrots, cucumbers, bell peppers, zucchini, and eggplant. Choose fruits and vegetables that are free from high FODMAP compounds like excess fructose or polyols.
- Protein Sources: Poultry (chicken, turkey), fish (salmon, cod, tuna), eggs, tofu, tempeh, and canned legumes like chickpeas and lentils (drained and rinsed to remove excess FODMAPs). Avoid marinades and sauces containing high FODMAP ingredients.
- Low FODMAP Dairy Alternatives: If lactose intolerance is a concern, stock up on lactose-free or dairy-free alternatives such as lactose-free milk, almond milk, rice milk, coconut milk, lactose-free yogurt, and lactose-free cheese. Choose unsweetened varieties to minimize added sugars.
- Herbs, Spices, and Flavorings: Spices, and seasonings like basil, oregano, parsley, thyme, rosemary, ginger, turmeric, cumin, paprika, mustard seeds, and vinegar except for apple cider vinegar. Avoid high FODMAP ingredients like onion and garlic powder, and opt for infused oils or garlic-infused oil for added flavor.

- Condiments and Sauces: Soy sauce (use tamari for gluten-free), Worcestershire sauce (check for gluten-free varieties), mustard, mayonnaise, ketchup (without high fructose corn syrup), olive oil, and balsamic vinegar.
- Snacks and Treats: Rice cakes, popcorn, rice crackers, gluten-free pretzels, nuts (in moderation), dark chocolate without added high FODMAP ingredients, and low FODMAP energy bars.
- Baking Essentials: If you enjoy baking, stock up on low FODMAP baking essentials like gluten-free flour blends (rice flour, oat flour, tapioca flour, potato starch), baking powder, baking soda, pure maple syrup, and vanilla extract. Try sweeteners like glucose, dextrose, or stevia.

SYMPTOMS TRACKING JOURNAL

DATE:
Meal/Recipe:

Put a check mark in the symptoms severity box

Symptoms	Mild	Moderate	Severe
Abdominal Pain			
Bloating			
Gas			
Diarrhoea			
Constipation			
Other Symptoms			

Notes/Comments

....

DATE:
Meal/Recipe:

Put a check mark in the symptoms severity box

Symptoms	Mild	Moderate	Severe
Abdominal Pain			
Bloating			
Gas			
Diarrhoea			
Constipation			
Other Symptoms			

Notes/Comments

DATE:
Meal/Recipe:

Put a check mark in the symptoms severity box

Symptoms	Mild	Moderate	Severe
Abdominal Pain			
Bloating			
Gas			
Diarrhoea			
Constipation			
Other Symptoms			

Notes/Comments

DATE:
Meal/Recipe:

Put a check mark in the symptoms severity box

Symptoms	Mild	Moderate	Severe
Abdominal Pain			
Bloating			
Gas			
Diarrhoea			
Constipation			
Other Symptoms			

Notes/Comments

....

DATE:
Meal/Recipe:

Put a check mark in the symptoms severity box

Symptoms	Mild	Moderate	Severe
Abdominal Pain			
Bloating			
Gas			
Diarrhoea			
Constipation			
Other Symptoms			

Notes/Comments

....

DATE:
Meal/Recipe:

Put a check mark in the symptoms severity box

Symptoms	Mild	Moderate	Severe
Abdominal Pain			
Bloating			
Gas			
Diarrhoea			
Constipation			
Other Symptoms			

Notes/Comments

....

DATE:
Meal/Recipe:

Put a check mark in the symptoms severity box

Symptoms	Mild	Moderate	Severe
Abdominal Pain			
Bloating			
Gas			
Diarrhoea			
Constipation			
Other Symptoms			

Notes/Comments

....

REINTRODUCTION SYMPTOMS ASSESSMENT

DATE:

Food/Ingredients to Reintroduce

Symptoms Assessment

Notes/Comments

DATE:

Food/Ingredients to Reintroduce

Symptoms Assessment

Notes/Comments

....

DATE:

Food/Ingredients to Reintroduce

Symptoms Assessment

Notes/Comments

....

DATE:

Food/Ingredients to Reintroduce

Symptoms Assessment

Notes/Comments

....

DATE:

Food/Ingredients to Reintroduce

Symptoms Assessment

Notes/Comments

....

DATE:

Food/Ingredients to Reintroduce

Symptoms Assessment

Notes/Comments

....

DATE:

Food/Ingredients to Reintroduce

Symptoms Assessment

Notes/Comments

....

Conversion Charts

Dry Ingredients

USA (Cups)	UK (Metric)
1 cup	240 ml
½ cup	120 ml
⅓ cup	80 ml
¼ cup	60 ml
1 tablespoon	15 ml
1 teaspoon	5 ml

Liquid Ingredients

USA (Fluid Ounces)	UK (Metric)
1 fluid ounce	30 ml
½ fluid ounce	15 ml
¼ fluid ounce	7.5 ml
⅛ ounce	3.75 ml
1 tablespoon	15 ml
1 teaspoon	5 ml

RECIPE INDEX

Almond Flour Blueberry Muffins 230
Baked Apples 228
Baked chicken breast and mashed sweet potatoes 205
Baked Chicken Breast and Sautéed Spinach 73
Baked Cod and Quinoa Pilaf 92
Baked cod and wild rice 209
Baked Potato and Steamed Broccoli 151
Baked salmon and quinoa 199
Baked Turkey Meatballs and Spaghetti Squash 114
Banana Nice Cream 218
Beef and Basmati Rice 147
Beef and Bean Chili 134
Beef with Broccoli 132
Beef and Cabbage Soup 141
Beef and Mushroom Stroganoff 139
Black Bean Tacos with Corn Tortillas 33
Caprese Salad with Tomato 45
Chia seed pudding with berries 194
Chickpea and Basmati Rice 83
Chickpea and Vegetable Curry 29
Chicken Caesar Salad and Dairy-Free Dressing 124
Chicken, Stir-Fry and Brown Rice 118
Chicken, Vegetable Stir-Fry and Brown Rice 71
Chicken with tamari sauce 192
Coconut Yogurt Parfait 222

Dark Chocolate 216
Eggplant and Zucchini Lasagna 95
Eggplant Parmesan and Vegan Cheese 51
Falafel Bowl and Mediterranean Salad 43
Greek yogurt parfait with berries 183
Grilled chicken and Roasted Potatoes 110
Grilled chicken salad and olive oil vinaigrette 174
Gluten-Free Pasta with Tomato Basil Sauce 88
Grilled Portobello Mushroom Burger 49
Grilled Salmon with Steamed Vegetables 67
Grilled shrimp skewers and marinara sauce 203
Grilled Steak and Mashed Sweet Potatoes 130
Grilled steak with roasted asparagus 207
Grilled Steak with Roasted Brussels Sprouts 81
Grilled Turkey Burger 122
Hasselback Potatoes with Rosemary 165
Hummus and Veggie Wrap 37
IBS Fruit Salad 214
Lamb Kebabs and Quinoa Tabbouleh 136
Lemon Herb Roasted Chicken Thighs 116
Lentil and vegetable soup 196
Lentil Soup and Spinach 27
Lentil Soup with Carrots and Kale 79
Mashed Potatoes 153
Meatloaf and Steamed Green Beans 145
Night Prepared Oats 176
Oatmeal Cookies 220
Omelet with mushrooms 187
Peanut Butter Energy Balls 226
Pork Stir-Fry with Bell Peppers 149
Pork Tenderloin with Roasted Root Vegetables 143
Potato and Leek Soup 161
Potato and Vegetable Frittata 169
Potato Pancakes 167
Potato Salad with Dijon Mustard Dressing 157
Quinoa and black bean salad 189

Quinoa Salad and Tahini Dressing 25
Quinoa salad with chickpeas 181

Quinoa Salad with Roasted Vegetables 69
Quinoa Stuffed Acorn Squash 64
Quinoa Stuffed Bell Peppers and Salsa 107
Rice Noodle and Soy Sauce 35
Rice Pudding 224
Roasted Potato Wedges and Herbs 155
Roasted Vegetable Pizza and Red Onion 60
Roasted Vegetable Salad and Balsamic Glaze 103
Scalloped Potatoes and Yeast 163
Scrambled eggs with spinach 172
Shrimp and Avocado Salad 75
Smoothie and protein powder 180
Smoothie bowl and pumpkin seeds 191
Spinach and Ricotta Stuffed Pasta Shells 53
Spinach with Gluten-Free Toast 97
Stir-fried tofu and brown rice 201
Stuffed Bell Peppers and Corn 39
Sweet Potato Hash with and Spinach 159
Tofu and Vegetable Pad Thai 99
Tofu Stir-Fry and Tamari Sauce 31
Turkey and avocado lettuce wraps 178
Turkey and Avocado Wrap 126
Turkey and Gluten-Free Tortilla 105
Turkey and Vegetable Chili 90
Turkey and Vegetable Kabobs 128
Turkey and Vegetable Soup 120
Turkey and vegetable soup 185
Turkey Chili and Crushed Tomatoes 112
Turkey meatballs and marinara sauce 211
Turkey Meatballs with Spaghetti Squash 77
Vegan Buddha Bowl and Tahini Sauce 101
Vegan Chili with Kidney Beans 41
Vegetable Frittata with Spinach 47
Vegetable Pad Thai with Tofu 55
Vegetable Stir-Fry with Broccoli 86
Vegetarian Sushi Rolls and Carrot 58

Veggie Wrap with Goat Cheese 62